Understanding Leaky Gut & Digestive Health

Simple Steps to Avoid Complications, Reduce Medical Expenses, Decrease Stress and Live a Healthy & Proactive Life

Dr. Ashley Sullivan, PharmD

Table of Contents

Introduction

As a child, I waged a relentless battle against my mother's attempts to conquer my aversion to vegetables and fruits. She tried a million different ways to get me to eat healthy food. I remember her saying, "You are what you eat," which often left me feeling confused. I questioned how on earth I could transform into a carrot or an apple simply by ingesting them. Perhaps you too have memories like this from your youth. Yet, even amidst my protests, my mother's recurring mantra remained an echo in my ears. Little did I know that over the years this seemingly simple phrase would unveil its profound truth.

Through a journey marked by trial and error, I discovered a revelation that transcends the whimsical notion of turning into a vegetable. I realized that we truly "are what we eat" because our gut only functions fully when it is fed well. The key then to a flourishing life lies in nurturing our gut—the epicenter of vitality.

In this book, I invite you to explore the transformative power that resides within the delicate ecosystem of our gut. Unveiling the secrets to fortifying it not only enhances our immune system but also acts as a catalyst for overall physical and mental well-being. Join me as we delve into the captivating world of gut health, where every morsel we consume becomes a brushstroke on the canvas of our inner vitality. It's time to repaint the story of our health, to embrace the symbiotic blending of our food and our gut.

Sandra's Story

Struggling with gut health has become extremely common, especially for women in middle age and above. I often see this both in my functional medicine practice and in my health coaching clients. Sandra, a forty-two-year-old woman, was caught in the whirlwind of life's demands, a familiar narrative for many women in middle age and beyond. As she navigated the challenges of being a devoted mother of three, her days were marked by the relentless grind of stressful, long work hours.

Sandra's demanding routine had become a breeding ground for chronic stress, a silent but potent disruptor of her gut health. The stressors in her life, stemming from both the responsibilities of motherhood and the pressures of her professional life, cast a shadow on her overall well-being. The impact of stress on her gut health was profound, as it triggered a cascade of physiological responses that threatened to compromise the delicate balance of her gut microbiome.

During this chaotic existence, Sandra found solace in quick, easy, and highly processed food options, further exacerbating her struggle with gut health. The convenience of these choices, while offering a momentary reprieve from her demanding schedule, set the stage for a host of digestive issues. Over time, the constant consumption of processed foods took a toll on her gut, leading to frequent stomach aches and discomfort.

As Sandra battled with her declining physical health, her mental well-being began to crumble under the weight of these stressors. This is because the intricate connection between the gut and the brain, often referred to as the gut-brain axis, plays a pivotal role in regulating mood and emotional responses. The turmoil in Sandra's gut health had started to manifest in her mental state, contributing to a decline in her overall mood and cognitive function.

Not only was Sandra's physical and mental health at stake but her family also began to witness the toll these struggles were taking on her life. Concerned for her well-being, they witnessed a woman they loved grappling with the complex interplay between stress, gut health, and mental health.

The repercussions extended beyond the realms of stress and gut health, reaching into Sandra's cardiovascular system. The chronic stress, coupled with poor dietary choices, resulted in elevated blood pressure levels. The intricate connection between gut health and blood pressure became evident as Sandra's physiological responses to stressors contributed to hypertension.

Sandra's story is an illustration of the intricate web woven between stress, gut health, and blood pressure. It reveals the importance of addressing the root causes of gut-related issues to achieve holistic well-being. Sandra's journey unveils the profound impact that lifestyle stressors can have on our body's intricate systems, which emphasizes the need for a comprehensive approach to health.

Jenny's Story

Next, we meet Jenny, a thirty-nine-year-old woman whose life took an unexpected turn when she found herself seeking care due to persistent stomach aches and bloating. A once vibrant and energetic individual, Jenny's complaint unveiled a cascade of health concerns that had insidiously crept into her daily life.

For several weeks, Jenny battled the discomfort of constant stomach aches and the frustrating sensation of bloating, both of which had become constant companions, overshadowing her ability to enjoy a proper meal. The toll on her physical appearance was evident. She had lost a significant amount of weight in an alarmingly short period, and her skin, once radiant, now bore premature wrinkles.

The impact wasn't merely skin-deep; Jenny's vitality was depleted, and lethargy became her unwelcome companion. Daily activities that were once second nature now became a huge effort, leaving her fatigued and drained. The vibrant woman who once effortlessly navigated her routine found herself grappling with a new reality, one that seemed to age her beyond her years.

As the symptoms persisted, so did Jenny's concern. Each passing day brought new worries, and the confusion around her declining health fueled her anxiety. Her apprehension intensified as her inability to carry out daily activities at an average pace increased, creating a perpetual cycle of physical discomfort and mental distress.

Jenny's journey, like Sandra's, also speaks to the intricate relationship between gut health and overall well-being. Her stomach aches and bloating are not just isolated symptoms; they are windows into a deeper imbalance within her gut microbiome. The repercussions extend far beyond mere digestive discomfort, permeating into her appearance, energy levels, and daily functionality.

As Jenny embarked on the path to seeking care, we peeled back the layers of her struggles to reveal the interconnectedness of gut health with various facets of our lives. It serves as an important reminder that the symptoms we experience are often manifestations of a broader health narrative. Jenny's story speaks to the importance of addressing gut health for a holistic and rejuvenated life.

Claire's Story

Let's delve into the life of Claire, a forty-seven-year-old woman whose health journey began when she found herself grappling with stomach ulcers that defied conventional treatment. The chronic nature of her condition weighed heavily on her, creating a deep sense of distress and concern for her overall well-being.

Claire, the accomplished director of a bustling marketing agency, unfolded a narrative woven with relentless work hours. Her daily grind extended between ten and fourteen hours, demanding her attention at least six days a week. In the chaotic rhythm of her professional life, convenience took precedence over nutrition. Claire found herself relying on processed foods and frequently resorting to fast food options and takeout meals, subjecting her stomach to a barrage of challenges.

This demanding professional life was not the sole contributor to Claire's health predicament. Her sedentary lifestyle, devoid of any form of physical activity, cast a shadow on her well-being. The consequence was evident—Claire found herself teetering on the brink of obesity, a stark manifestation of the toll her work-centric routine had taken on her body.

As her stomach ulcers persisted, so did the emotional turmoil within Claire. The realization that conventional medications were falling short of alleviating her condition heightened her anxiety. Concerns about her health began to permeate every facet of her life, adversely affecting her professional achievements and personal happiness.

Claire's story is a stark reminder of the complex dance between lifestyle choices, gut health, and overall well-being. The ulcers in her stomach were not isolated incidents but rather signals of an internal imbalance exacerbated by her relentless work schedule, poor dietary choices, and lack of physical activity.

As Claire stood at the crossroads of her health journey, the imperative for change became evident. Claire grappled with the urgent need to make amends to her lifestyle. Her symptoms were a call to action, not only to treat her ulcers but to reclaim control over her health and enhance the quality of her life.

In the arc of Claire's narrative, we witness the transformative potential that lies in acknowledging the symbiotic relationship between gut health, lifestyle, and overall well-being.

The Common Denominator

In all three circumstances, the underlying cause was the lack of a healthy, well-functioning gut microbiome (bacterial flora). A common misconception is that eating only green vegetables is the key to "being healthy." However, we need proper nourishment from various kinds of foods to lead an active and healthy life.

More than 60 million people alone in the US suffer from issues related to the gut, such as irritable bowel syndrome and inflammatory bowel disease. Some of these typical issues are bloating, diarrhea, stomach discomfort, gas, migraines, and auto-immune diseases. People have also commonly complained about having mood swings, developing allergies, weight loss/gain, and having food cravings (often related to eating a high processed sugar diet).

When experiencing such issues, people often worry about what they're eating and if eating a certain food will cause their health to worsen. The constant worry and regulation of their symptoms can cause them to have anxiety and mental stress.

Are you going through something similar? Do you feel like you can relate to the symptoms above? Have you also been trying various household remedies and supplements that promise a healthier gut, but to no avail? Are you tired of people giving you unsolicited advice to treat your stomach bloating?

If your response to these questions is "YES," then you have picked up the right book! It will answer all your questions and get you on the proper track to treat your gut.

But how? Well, simply because this book has been carefully researched and thoroughly compiled by me, a practicing pharmacist with a strong interest in holistic and functional medicine. My comprehensive study in medicine has allowed me to understand what type of medicine works best for a particular condition. In addition, I am a wellness advocate and an integrative health coach and have treated people with digestive imbalances. As a female medical practitioner, I have paid particular attention to women who are undergoing digestive issues. These often cause hormone imbalances, particularly when those women have become too lenient with what they are consuming on a long-term basis. With this first-hand knowledge of digestive issues, I intend to empower my readers with knowledge about their digestive system and the importance it plays in their health.

The book is divided into eight chapters. These will thoroughly explain the function of the gut, and the real-life impact when it's not taken care of, helping you to understand the gut's needs and what works best for it, and giving testimonies of people who have had issues with a bad gut and how they were able to treat it with my help.

As I have gathered from my experience, it is exceedingly difficult to achieve the right results unless you have accurate information and methods to do it. So, our journey does not end in gaining more knowledge and understanding; at the back of the book, I have included some delicious and healthy recipes to help maintain optimal gut function.

Join us in this journey of discovery and equip yourself with more knowledge about your gut and digestive system. You can make informed choices on the foods you should eat and changes you can make to your lifestyle. Your future self will thank you for making this investment in yourself. Turn the page and take the first step toward a healthy digestive system!

CHAPTER ONE

The Marvels of Digestion

M eet Emma, a vibrant woman in her mid-thirties who is juggling the demands of her paralegal job at a law firm with studying for law exams. One evening, while having dinner, she was blindsided by a sudden bout of severe and persistent diarrhea. Feeling embarrassed and scared, she decided to seek help at the hospital. Little did she know, this was just the beginning of a health rollercoaster.

Soon after, Emma found herself grappling with stomach aches, bloating, gas, and a newfound intolerance to certain foods. Concerned about her health, she embarked on a quest to understand her symptoms, consulting doctors and medical experts. The toll on her energy levels and her ability to complete daily tasks became overwhelming as her health rapidly declined.

A diagnosis revealed Leaky Gut Syndrome, a condition where her intestinal lining had become permeable, allowing toxins and bacteria to escape into her bloodstream. With a tailored diet and medication, Emma reclaimed her health, returning to her routine worry-free and embracing a healthy life once again. Emma's journey highlights the importance of gut health, demonstrating both how it impacts our daily lives and the transformative power of proper care and attention.

Just like Emma, millions of people undergo stomach issues regularly. The reason that it's so prevalent is that most people don't have the required knowledge to diagnose their issues and don't understand the role that our gut plays in maintaining our body. Hence why it's imperative to know how our digestion works and ways to nourish it.

Why is Healthy Digestion so Important?

Food is our body's fuel. We need it to conduct various tasks throughout the day. When food is consumed, the process of digestion breaks it down into a form that can be stored inside the human body.

But what happens when our body is not performing digestion properly? What happens when the food won't break down into a million pieces for digestion?

As we have seen in the featured case studies, we can undergo a multitude of issues that cause hindrances in our daily lives. While it's common to experience some temporary digestive issues occasionally, it's not okay to have these frequently. Some of the recurrent issues I'm referring to are heartburn, diarrhea, constipation, hemorrhoids, gastroenteritis, ulcers, and gallstones. Even though some of these are temporary, they can be quite painful if not treated on time with the proper procedure.

However, sometimes people also develop diseases related to the digestive tissues, which can often remain for a lifetime and prove to be detrimental to health. Some examples are gastroesophageal reflux disease, irritable bowel syndrome, lactose intolerance, diverticulosis, diverticulitis, Crohn's disease, celiac disease, and even cancer. It's crucial to make sure that your gut remains healthy.

But how do we know if our gut is healthy or not? Is there a way to know that?

Overview of the Digestive System

In a healthy digestive system, all the digestive enzymes and juices are produced and used in the right amounts, the good intestinal bacteria are there to be used, the nutrients are absorbed, elimination of pathogenic bacteria occurs, and toxins and waste from the gut are removed. Let's look at a case study of Lindsey to see how an ideal digestive system should be.

Case Study

Lindsey is a thirty-five-year-old accountant who's mastered the art of maintaining a healthy digestive system. She's not your average number cruncher; Lindsey takes a thoughtful approach to her well-being. When it comes to groceries, she's like a detective, meticulously scanning labels so that she can make informed choices to keep sugars and fats in check. Lindsey knows that as she gracefully ages, it's crucial to treat her digestive system with some extra TLC.

Her mornings kick off with a burst of energy, thanks to a thirty-minute yoga session, and she seamlessly integrates gym workouts every two days to stay fit. Lindsey doesn't just balance her books; she's also a pro at managing stress. Recognizing its potential impact on her mental and physical health, she tackles stress head-on, ensuring it doesn't linger.

But that's not all–Lindsey's dedication to digestive health goes beyond the gym. She also keeps a watchful eye on her bowel movements, making sure they maintain a consistent frequency. I want to encourage you that Lindsey's story is an achievable journey of mindful eating, staying active, and managing stress. The advice you'll read in this book can become the blueprint you follow when you begin to prioritize your digestive well-being in the hustle and bustle of everyday life.

Keeping Track of Bowel Movements

You can figure out if all the processes in your gut are being carried out accurately by keeping track of your bowel movements. A healthy person usually takes up to 24-25 hours to completely digest food and expel the waste products from the body. Note the time it took for you to pass out your stool, along with how it looked, to figure out if your body is working properly.

I understand that it can be uncomfortable to talk about the passage of your stool and its appearance, even with a medical practitioner. However, it's important to have this basic knowledge about your stool to check if your gut is working properly.

A normal stool should, ideally, be four to eight inches long, like a log or a cylinder in appearance. If it's coming out in pellets, it's not normal and means that you may have constipation. Conversely, if it's too runny, you have diarrhea. It should look firm and soft. If it was easy to pass out without any major force, then it lies under that description.

In addition, the color of the stool should be brown, with light and darker shades included. Brown is the color of bile, so having a large area of brown is completely normal. If your stool looks green, it's usually okay and can often be because of dietary choices, such as the inclusion of a lot of green vegetables in your food or even the addition of artificial color if it's too green (such as blue cupcake icing!). Medications, such as antibiotics and iron supplements, may also cause green-colored stool. Red, however, can be concerning since it might mean that your colon is bleeding. If you see red in your stool, visit a medical practitioner. Yellow stool is often stinky and can mean that you either have too much fat in your diet or that your food is not being absorbed properly. Whereas a pale white stool can mean that you have some sort of infection.

Moreover, you should only take a few minutes to pass out the stool. If it takes you more than ten to fifteen minutes, it means that you have constipation and lack fiber in your diet. Nutritional sources of fiber include whole grains (brown rice, quinoa, oats, whole wheat bread), legumes (beans, chickpeas, peas), fruit (apples, pears, berries, oranges, bananas), vegetables (broccoli, carrots, brussels sprouts, cauliflower, leafy greens), nuts and seeds, dried fruits, popcorn, and bran cereal. There is no fixed number of times you should be passing stools in a day. It's perfectly normal to pass feces as much as three times a day or as little as three times a week. The essential thing is that you have your own 'normal' pattern of bowel movement.

The Main Organs Involved in the Digestive System

Digestion is a complex process, so before we can talk about how to fix your digestive issues, we need to understand digestion in detail, including how nutrients are absorbed in your body. The main organs that take part are the mouth, esophagus, stomach, pancreas, liver, gallbladder, small intestine, large intestine (colon), and anus. Even before we start eating, the mouth anticipates food, beginning the process of digestion through the creation of saliva and the salivary enzyme known as salivary amylase. This is one of the first enzymes to encounter food as your body begins the process of breaking it down.

Your tongue pushes the food down into your throat, through the esophagus, and into the stomach. The stomach then mixes the food with the various digestive enzymes, until the food is a semi-liquid mixture called chyme. Peristaltic motion helps the mixture slowly release into the small intestine. Once there, the liver, pancreas, and intestines use their digestive enzymes to enhance the process of digestion, readying the food for absorption.

The digestive system is a complex network of nine organs that work together to break down food, absorb nutrients, and eliminate waste. Each organ plays a specific role in this process, ensuring that the body receives the necessary nutrients for energy, growth, and maintenance.

How Does the Gut Absorb Nutrients?

Thousands of small projections lining the small intestine absorb the nutrients, before releasing them into the bloodstream to be used and stored. Water is also absorbed into the small intestine through diffusion into the bloodstream, which is why it's important to drink eight to ten glasses a day to stay hydrated. At the same time, waste products are transferred to the large intestine and into the rectum to be removed.

In addition to the enzymes and digestive juices in the stomach and small intestine, there are gut bacteria called microbes in the large intestine and colon that help to digest food. In total, there are around 100 trillion microbes in your gut, separated into two types: good and bad. The good microbes are known as symbiotic, and the bad bacteria are called pathogens. What we eat determines the benefit or damage our intestine receives. Good bacteria are important in the digestion of macronutrients—like fats, carbohydrates, proteins—and micronutrients, which include vitamins and minerals. After the indigestible nutrients enter the large intestine, the microbes help ferment the remaining proteins and carbohydrates, producing short-chain fatty acids, known as SCFA, which are used as fuel for tasks in the body.

How is Food Digested in the Body?

Let's say you had a chicken sandwich for lunch. Did you get all the basic nutrients for the day? A chicken sandwich primarily includes proteins coming from the chicken, carbohydrates provided by the bread, fiber from any vegetables that might be present in the sandwich, fats from mayonnaise, cheese, butter (or if any oil was used while cooking the chicken), and vitamins, such as vitamins A and B. Proteins are broken down into amino acids, carbohydrates into simple sugars, and fats into glycerol. The different nutrients are broken down by the organs assigned to that task and stored in the body for use in the next few hours of your day.

The carbohydrates found in the bread provide immediate energy, taking only fifteen minutes to three hours to be absorbed. The fat source found in dairy products (mayonnaise and cheese) absorbs quickly into the body, taking between thirty minutes to two hours to be fully digested. Fiber-containing vegetables and fruits, meanwhile, take a while longer (almost a whole day) to be absorbed. At almost three days, the protein source found in the chicken takes the longest to absorb.

Have you ever noticed that eating certain kinds of food causes you discomfort, for example, spicy food? It's because some foods are easily absorbed by the body, giving you proper energy from the nutrients, while some make your digestive system work harder. Spicy food, like hot chili peppers; fatty foods, such as red meat; fried food, such as french fries; and acidic foods are more difficult for the body to absorb. In contrast, chicken, eggs, salmon, sweet potatoes, bananas, and rice are easily digested by the human body. This is why most nutrition should come from lean meats, fruits, vegetables, and whole grains.

How Modern Life Puts Our Digestive System at Risk

Our daily life has become so busy that there's barely any time to put effort into what we eat, and we usually end up eating what is convenient: a meal from a fast-food restaurant or packaged processed food. This unhealthy eating leads us to eventually reduce the diversity of foods we consume. According to a study (McDonald et. al, 2018), people who consumed more than thirty types of plant-based food in a week had a wider variety of microbes in their bodies in comparison with those who didn't. This study shows that it's necessary to diversify your foods because microbes are an essential part of digestion.

Additionally, because our lives have become hectic and spending time on ourselves is considered a luxury, we usually don't find the time and energy to commit to exercising daily. However, physical fitness is important; it not only increases the good bacteria in the gut but also helps elevate mood and decrease stress levels.

We have become too involved in the 'grind' that tells us to keep working without any rest. This causes our stress levels to rise, which in turn increases alcohol consumption and encourages indulging in cigarette smoking. These habits eventually cause the body to get sicker, further increasing the use of antibiotics—a huge contributing factor in the destruction of gut bacteria and, ultimately, the destruction of health.

Not taking care of the gut also means fewer enzymes in the body for digestion. Read on further to see how important enzymes are in the digestive process.

The Role of Enzymes and the Digestive System

What are enzymes exactly, and why are they so important? The simple answer is that enzymes are catalysts that speed up the digestion process, without which food will not be broken down the way it needs to be. Carbohydrates need the enzyme amylase to be broken down, whereas proteins require protease, and fats need lipase.

Enzyme Deficiency

A reduction in these enzymes can hinder proper digestion and cause several enzyme deficiencies, such as food intolerance, digestive issues, poor nutrient absorption, weight gain, a poorer immune system, fatigue and lethargy, anxiety and depression, and skin problems.

People who do not consciously take notice of the food they are eating can often develop enzyme deficiency, in addition to having lower microbes in the body. One example is John, a thirty-eight-year-old engineer who suffers from enzyme deficiency due to a genetic predisposition. This condition has an uncomfortable impact on his digestion, inducing cramps, bloating, and nutrient absorption problems. He has to take certain enzyme supplements to aid in digestion and be very careful about his diet. Some enzyme deficiencies are more common in women than in men, such as lactose intolerance. Women, especially, are at a higher risk of developing osteoporosis than men; hence, they need to get enough vitamin C and calcium.

Some enzyme deficiencies are more prevalent in certain areas. This is known as the cultural enzymatic effect. The prevalence of lactose intolerance, for example, has a geographical variation. Studies have shown that it is more widespread in Asia, Africa, the Middle East, and Latin America. Other regions where milk was made a mandatory part of daily diet several thousand years ago developed lactase persistence due to the prevalence of lactose in their diet, and, as a result, these populations can now absorb lactose easily (Anguita-Ruiz 2020).

The Gut Microbiome

The human gut is inhabited by trillions of microorganisms known as the microbiome, which consists of bacteria, fungi, and viruses. They play a very crucial part in the maintenance of the digestive system and overall physical and mental health, affecting the absorption and even the mood of an individual. Gut microbes can be maintained by diet and regular exercise.

The Importance of a Balanced Gut Microbiome

A balanced gut microbiome is essential for the well-being of the digestive system. It makes sure that digestion is efficient, supports the immune system, and encourages good mental health. It also aids weight management through keeping inflammation under control and increasing nutrient absorption. A good microbiome is responsible for preventing disease development, keeping the gut-brain connection healthy, and maintaining healthy metabolism. Maintaining a balanced gut microbiome is an integral part of having a healthy life.

What are Prebiotics, Probiotics, and Postbiotics?

The three "biotics" work in a cyclic manner. Prebiotics are the source of fuel for probiotics and usually take the form of food we eat, such as apples, asparagus, barley, and wheat. Probiotics are the living bacteria in the gut that feed on prebiotics. And postbiotics, such as butyrate, are what the probiotics produce to help regulate the gut environment, which eventually lowers inflammation in the gut.

Gut Wisdom Challenge!
How Well Do You Know Your Digestive System?

- What is the main function of the small intestine in the gut?

1. Storing food

2. Absorbing nutrients

3. Removing Toxins

- Probiotics are good for your health.

1. True

2. False

- How many microbes are there in your gut?

1. 10 billion

2. 10 trillion

3. 100 trillion

- What's the recommended daily water intake for an adult?

1. 1-2 glasses

2. 4-6 glasses

3. 8-10 glasses

- Which of the below organs is not part of the digestive system?

1. Pancreas

2. Lungs

3. Liver

- How many organs are in the digestive system?

1. 3

2. 5

3. 7

4. 9

- Which of these is a good source of fiber content for the body?

1. Sugary cereal

2. White bread

3. Broccoli

- Is physical exercise necessary to maintain your gut health?

1. Yes

2. No

- What is the process called where food breaks down into a semi-liquid mixture called chyme in the stomach?

1. Digestion

2. Peristalsis

3. Absorption

(Answers: 2,1,3,3,2,4,3,1,1)

I hope this chapter helped you understand your digestive system better. However, we have only uncovered the tip of the iceberg here; the digestive system is much more intricate than this. As we continue reading, we will explore its inner workings and its role in our health.

Now that we know how it all works, what happens if it stops working the way it should? How does our body react then? Read on to find the answers to these questions and more.

CHAPTER TWO

Unraveling Digestive Disorders

S o far, 88.99 million lives have been completely altered by digestive diseases, to the extent that they reduced the person's life expectancy. The disability-adjusted life years (DALYs) formula calculates the number of life years lost due to ill-health in comparison with a healthy life span. It ranks digestive issues in thirteenth place as the cause of DALYs globally. Cirrhosis and liver diseases prevail more than others. Geographically, South Asia is disproportionally affected by digestive issues over other regions (Wang et. al, 1990).

These alarming statistics call for us to prioritize our gut health so that we may live a prosperous life. However, we can only treat them once we understand how they affect our gut. This chapter will discuss various gut issues and their underlying causes, symptoms, and possible treatments.

The Main Gut Issues

As the statistics suggest, digestive issues have been increasing at an accelerated rate. Let's take Sara, for example. In her early forties, she was dealing with a hiatal hernia. This is caused by a small hole in the diaphragm, which the stomach then pushes through. She commonly felt heartburn, especially if she had consumed too many spices in her food. She also felt that sometimes her food was coming back up in her mouth. In addition, she also experienced chest pain and difficulty swallowing. Since she was also borderline obese, the increased pressure in her abdomen worsened her condition. She was advised to make amends to her routine, eat healthily, and do some physical exercise to keep the symptoms as minimal as possible. Surgery would be considered if the situation didn't improve.

Jasmine, on the other hand, also a middle-aged woman, had colon polyps, a condition in which cells start forming on the lining of the intestine. Her uncle had colon cancer in his later years, so there was a possibility that this was driven by a genetic predisposition. She used to be a smoker as well, which adds to the risk factors but quit when she realized she was in danger of developing cancer. She will soon undergo surgery to remove the colon polyps before there is any chance that they mature into cancer.

Hiatal hernia and colon polyps are just two of the widespread digestive issues witnessed regularly. The table below highlights more recurrent gut issues, detailing what they are, their causes, the common symptoms observed, and what one must do and avoid reducing further issues.

Digestive issue	What it is	Causes	Symptoms	Do's	Don'ts
Constipation	Unable to pass stool regularly	• Lack of fiber in the diet • Change in routine • Medication side effects • Not hydrated enough	• Stomach cramps • Feeling bloated • Feeling sick • Loss of appetite	• Take 18-30g of fiber a day • Eat fruits and vegetables • Exercise regularly • Take prescribed laxatives	• Eat processed food • Add fiber too fast and in sudden large quantities • Drink alcohol • Consume too much dairy
Diarrhea	Watery stool and frequent bowel movements	• Viruses (Coronavirus, Rotavirus, Norwalk virus, etc.) • Bacteria and parasites (E. coli, Clostridiumoides difficile) • Medications, such as antibiotics • Lactose intolerance	• Stomach cramps • Bloating • Nausea • Vomiting • Fever • Blood in stool • Urgent need to empty bowels	• Drink more water to stay hydrated • Take prescribed anti-diarrheal medicine • Take probiotics	• Eat high-fiber or oily/fatty foods • Workout extensively • Consume alcohol or hot beverages • Eat dairy for a while
Colon Polyps	Cells start lining the colon. They can cause cancer over time	• Change in genes can cause the production of cells even when they are not needed, causing polyps to form • Polyps are nonneoplastic (non-cancerous) and neoplastic (can become cancerous)	Initially, polyps might not show any symptoms. However, the common ones are: • Long-lasting diarrhea or constipation • Blood in stool • Anemia • Abdominal pain • Rectal bleeding • Dizziness	• Eat less meat • Eat more fruits and vegetables • Regular exercise • Lose weight if you're overweight	• Consume alcohol • Smoke • Eat fatty foods

Perianal abscesses / hemorrhoids / fissures	Collection of pus near the anus. While they are very painful, they do not affect the absorption of nutrients. It may be red in color and warm to touch.	• A tear in the anal canal • Sexually transmitted infection • Blocked anal glands • Diabetes, diverticulitis, colitis, being the recipient of anal sex, and pelvic inflammatory disease can increase the risk	• Constant, throbbing pain • Release of pus • Swelling, redness, and tenderness around the anus • Constipation • Fever • Chills • Malaise	• Stay hydrated • Have a sitz bath • Act on your bowel movement urges immediately • Use stool softeners or laxatives (prescribed) • Sleep well	• Eat fatty foods • Become constipated • Increase stress

Lactose intolerance	Inability to digest sugar in milk / dairy.	• Lack of production of enzyme lactase in small intestine • Risk factors include increasing age, premature birth, ethnicity and race (Native Americans, Hispanic, Asians and Africans are more prone), cancer treatments, surgery or disease, and small intestinal diseases)	• Bloating • Gas • Diarrhea • Nausea (sometimes vomiting too) • Stomach cramps (All these occur after consumption of milk or dairy)	• Consume lactose-free dairy products • Eat active culture foods, such as yogurt • Use substitutes for dairy, such as soy milk • Eat more vegetables and fruits to get calcium, such as broccoli, fish, tofu, and soybeans • Take lactase tablets	• Consume high-lactase products, such as cheese or butter in large amounts

Hiatal Hernia	The abdomen and diaphragm get separated by a bulge in the stomach. A small hernia is usually harmless. However, larger ones can cause food and acid to go back into the esophagus	• Changes in diaphragm due to age • An injury in the area • Having a large hiatus by birth • Constant intense pressure on the surrounding muscles from lifting weights, vomiting, or forceful bowel movements	• Heartburn • Pain in chest or abdomen • Acid reflux • Bloating • Shortness of breath • Passing black stool • Blood in vomit • Difficulty in swallowing food	• Eat low-fat dairy • Stay hydrated • Eat smaller and more frequent meals • Eat low-fat meals, such as lean chicken and fish • Add more grains (such as bran and oatmeal), beans, broccoli, and carrots to your diet	• Eat spicy food • Drink coffee • Eat dairy products • Eat fatty foods • Eat onions and garlic (they can cause heartburn) • Eat carbonated drinks • Eat or drink citrus fruits

In addition to the above-mentioned digestive issues, there are several more that are important to know about. As I frequently deal with patients with a variety of issues, I have noticed that certain conditions make people more prone to digestive issues.

Gastroesophageal Reflux Disease

Gastroesophageal reflux is a common disease in which it feels like food and stomach acid are moving out of the stomach through the mouth. In this condition, the person experiences heartburn, acid reflux, and abdominal pain, among other symptoms.

Case Study

Emily dealt with a common pregnancy-related issue—gastroesophageal reflux (GERD), particularly in her second trimester. As the baby's weight increased, the muscles around her lower esophagus did not relax how they needed to, sometimes causing stomach acid to come up to her throat. She constantly felt heartburn, had trouble swallowing, coughed, and felt nausea.

Her symptoms were not too severe, and her condition was easily diagnosed and monitored with diet changes. However, if the acid reflux is to such an extent that it may cause concern for esophageal health, and initial medication fails to work, there might be a need to perform a proper diagnosis using an upper endoscopy and reflux testing. The risk of having GERD increases if you are obese, pregnant, have connective tissue disorders, smoke, have an unhealthy eating routine and diet, and consume too much alcohol or coffee.

How to Manage Heartburn through Lifestyle Changes

Fortunately, GERD can be treated with a change in lifestyle if the symptoms aren't severe. Avoiding fried and fatty foods and carbonated drinks, exercising regularly to keep yourself physically active, and reducing weight if you're overweight, combined with making sure that you stop eating two to three hours before you lie down are ways to prevent GERD. Just following these three tips can be life-changing!

Decoding Your Gastroesophageal Reflux Disease

The different techniques to keep GERD at bay are as individual as the person experiencing them; there isn't one way that works for everyone. Henry, an accountant, had to make a minor shift in his pillow angle, elevating it a little, adjust his diet, and decide to avoid his trigger foods to lessen his GERD symptoms.

Penny, on the other hand, found some low-acid recipes and chose to experiment with those to see if they would help her acid reflux. To her delight, they did.

Molly, a yoga instructor, devised a yoga plan for herself, carefully choosing the postures that would help her stomach. Everyone's lifestyle and risk factors are different; find what works in your life.

Bloating: Causes and Remedies

Abdominal bloating, characterized by discomfort and a sense of fullness in the belly, can arise from various factors, including gas, fluid retention, irritable bowel syndrome (IBS), food intolerances, menstrual symptoms, and infections. While some instances can be self-managed, certain causes may necessitate medical attention.

Most often, though, it's attributed to indigestion or the accumulation of gas. Typically, it's not a cause for concern if it's linked to food consumption, does not worsen progressively, and resolves within a day or two.

Common causes encompass:

- *Gas:* The build-up of gas in the stomach and intestines manifests as symptoms like frequent burping, excessive gas, and an urgent need for bowel movement. Triggers may include specific foods or the ingestion of air.

- *Indigestion*: Discomfort or pain in the stomach, possibly accompanied by bloating, commonly results from overeating, excessive alcohol intake, or certain medications.

- *Infection:* Stomach infections, indicated by bloating in conjunction with symptoms like diarrhea, vomiting, nausea, and stomach pain. Bacterial or viral infections may be contributing factors.

- *Small Intestinal Bacterial Overgrowth (SIBO):* Imbalance in gut bacteria leading to chronic symptoms like bloating, frequent diarrhea, and challenges in digestion and nutrient absorption.

- *Fluid Retention:* Triggered by factors such as the consumption of salty foods, hormonal fluctuations, or food intolerances, resulting in heightened fluid retention. Persistent fluid-related bloating may signal underlying concerns like liver or kidney issues.

- *Food Intolerances:* Bloating may ensue after the consumption of specific foods, as seen in lactose intolerance, gluten intolerance, or celiac disease. Eliminating the problematic food source can alleviate symptoms.

In instances where bloating persists, is accompanied by alarming symptoms, or is associated with chronic conditions, seeking guidance from a healthcare professional is imperative. Additionally, if bloating coincides with fever, bloody stool, severe vomiting, or prolonged symptoms, consulting a medical professional is advisable.

Tips for Relieving Constipation

Relieving constipation often involves lifestyle changes and simple interventions. Here are some tips that may help:

Increase Fiber Intake: Consume more fiber-rich foods, such as fruits, vegetables, whole grains, and legumes. Gradually introduce fiber to your diet to avoid bloating or gas. Aim for at least twenty-five to thirty grams of fiber per day.

Stay Hydrated: Drink plenty of water throughout the day to soften stools and aid in digestion. Limit caffeine and alcohol intake, as they can contribute to dehydration.

Regular Physical Activity: Engage in regular exercise to stimulate bowel movements and promote overall digestive health. Even a short daily walk can be beneficial.

Include Probiotics: Consume probiotic-rich foods, like yogurt, or take probiotic supplements to promote a healthy gut microbiome.

Prunes and Fiber-Rich Foods: Prunes (dried plums) are a natural remedy for constipation. They contain both fiber and a natural laxative. Include other fiber-rich foods like bran cereal or oatmeal in your diet.

Limit Processed Foods: Reduce the intake of processed and low-fiber foods, as they can contribute to constipation.

Consider Natural Laxatives: Certain foods, like flaxseeds, chia seeds, and aloe vera, may have natural laxative effects. Be cautious with over-the-counter laxatives and consult a healthcare professional before using them regularly.

Warm Beverages: Warm liquids, such as herbal tea or warm water with lemon, can stimulate bowel movements (Meacham, n.d.).

If constipation persists or becomes a recurring issue, it's essential to consult with a healthcare provider to rule out any underlying conditions and determine an appropriate course of action. They can provide personalized advice based on your health and medical history.

Managing Diarrhea with Proper Hydration and Diet

Consuming bland foods, particularly those included in the BRAT diet (bananas, rice, applesauce, toast), can expedite the resolution of diarrhea and alleviate stomach discomfort.

Here are some tips to manage diarrhea through dietary choices:

Foods to Include in a Bland Diet:

- BRAT diet includes bananas, white rice, applesauce, and white bread toast.

- Additional options: cooked cereals, soda crackers, low-sugar apple juice, boiled potatoes.

BRAT Diet Benefits:

- These foods are bland and low in fiber, aiding in stool firming.

- Accelerates recovery from diarrhea.

- Prevents stomach upset and irritation.

Diet-Diarrhea Connection:

- Diarrhea causes vary, and can include allergies, food poisoning, or chronic conditions like irritable bowel syndrome.

- Long-term digestive conditions can be influenced by your food choices.

- Certain foods can either help restore digestive balance or worsen symptoms during episodes of diarrhea.

Hydration Importance:
- Stay hydrated to replace lost fluids during diarrhea.

- Recommended liquids: water, clear broths (without grease), electrolyte-enhanced water, weak tea.

Post-Recovery Food Introduction:
- Gradually reintroduce foods like scrambled eggs and cooked vegetables as recovery progresses (Seitz, 2023).

Gallstones

Another prominent digestive issue, particularly experienced by women, is the presence of gallstones. When cholesterol gathers inside the gallbladder, it hardens. This can cause pain in the upper-right abdomen or the center of the stomach. Even though the pain typically lasts a few hours, it can be very severe. In most cases, the gallbladder has to be removed through surgery so that the symptoms don't increase. If the surgery is not performed correctly, the person can experience high temperature, chills, nausea and vomiting, accelerated heartbeat, pale-yellow and itchy skin, loss of appetite, and diarrhea.

People who are obese and above the age of forty need to be especially careful with their lifestyle so that they don't suffer from gallstones. To avoid the risk, you must include healthy fats in your diet, such as fish and olive oil, remove processed sugars and fried foods, stay hydrated, and hit the treadmill occasionally.

Celiac Disease / Gluten Intolerance

As we delve further into studying digestive issues, let's discuss gluten intolerance and celiac disease. If you think the two diseases are the same, you are not the only one. It's not uncommon to presume so. In this section, I will help to clear up the differences between the two.

People with gluten intolerance get sick after ingesting gluten (a protein found in grains such as wheat and barley) and endure symptoms such as nausea, feeling tired, and bloated.

On the contrary, celiac disease is an autoimmune disease where the body fights against gluten as if it's a virus, causing inflammation and probable damage to the digestive tissues. Gluten intolerance can develop at any time in a person's life—some might even be born with it. Whereas people with Celiac disease have an abnormal gene in their body, along with an innumerable number of certain antibodies that fight gluten. Gluten intolerance is much more frequent, affecting 6 percent of the US population. Conversely, celiac disease affects 1 percent of the US population.

While gluten intolerance and celiac disease have their roots in different bodily systems, they both have similar symptoms. For those who experience either, a shift to gluten-free products, like gluten-free flour, is necessary. Exceptional care needs to be taken to not ingest any gluten so that symptoms don't worsen.

Even though there is no cure for the two diseases, keeping the symptoms at bay is easy: don't consume gluten! Yes, it might seem like an incredulous thought at first that you won't be eating wheat. However, gluten-free wheat and flour are readily available in stores and can be used as substitutes. Using gluten-free flour and substitutes such as oats, cornstarch, and nutmeg may help control symptoms. It certainly does not mean you have to restrict dining out. You can find some fun and easy recipes using gluten-free flour so that your taste buds don't have to compromise. All that's required is a little determination on your part!

Irritable Bowel Syndrome

Another conventional digestive issue is IBS (irritable bowel syndrome), which affects 10-15 percent of the adult population in the US. IBS is a mixture of many symptoms, most commonly constituting bloating, abdominal pain, constipation or diarrhea (or switching between the two), excess gas, and mucus in stool. Most often, the syndrome is found in women anytime from their teens to their late forties. Usually, certain foods and mental stress can trigger the symptoms.

Each person may have a different experience and list of symptoms with their IBS. Nevertheless, I can impart some basic knowledge about the kinds of foods you must eat if you are suffering with IBS. First and foremost, drink plenty of water, limit caffeine, and remove dairy products from your diet (since IBS patients are more prone to lactose intolerance). Also, increase your daily fiber intake. Hopefully, these few changes will help in the management of your IBS.

Rare and Complex Gut Issues

While the digestive issues discussed above are manageable and prove to be non-threatening to life in most cases, the gut has its complications. Sometimes, there can be severe and complex issues as well, which can be difficult to control with lifestyle changes and may require surgery.

Crohn's Disease and Ulcerative Colitis

One of these rare diseases is inflammatory bowel disease (IBD). Crohn's disease and ulcerative colitis also come under IBD. While the former can cause inflammation in any part of the gastrointestinal tract, the latter only occurs in the large intestine. However, both exhibit similar symptoms.

The customary diagnoses for these two diseases are blood tests, stool tests, endoscopies, and bowel imaging and scanning. Even though there is currently no cure for IBD, it can be treated with medication, lifestyle changes, surgery, and complementary and alternative medicine. If the directions are followed thoroughly, someone affected with the disease can live a fully productive life.

Case Study

Natalie, now thirty-four, was diagnosed with Crohn's disease nearly a decade ago and suffers from acute symptoms. Most commonly, she experiences inflammation in her small intestine, which causes her to experience harsh abdominal pain, diarrhea, fluctuation in her body weight, and pain in her joints. Moreover, her entire mood is also affected by her health. She was directed to make certain lifestyle changes, such as maintaining a diet rich in fiber and protein—which helped to give her a lot of energy—adding vitamins as supplements and exercising regularly. Medications, such as steroids, immunosuppressants, and antibiotics, are often used to manage this disease.

Gastroparesis

As we continue talking about chronic gut issues, gastroparesis cannot go unnoticed. The disease was discovered in 1958 by a doctor called Richard Kassander who observed something unusual while examining diabetic patients. He discovered that many of them were experiencing gastrointestinal issues such as nausea, vomiting, bloating, and feeling full quickly, even if their blood sugar levels were acceptable. He was intrigued and decided to investigate further.

Kassander discovered that all these stomach ailments were related to one thing: their stomachs were taking longer than usual to empty after eating. The delay in emptying was generating their suffering (Surtini 2021). This discovery was significant because it was the first time anyone had detected this problem in diabetics. He named it diabetic gastroparesis.

More recently, a study was conducted on a forty-six-year-old man who had been vomiting for five months when he was eventually admitted to Queen Elizabeth Central Hospital. He would vomit at least five times a day and complained of constipation. Apart from being diagnosed with diabetes mellitus 2, there were no other possible causes that were found (Zhang et. al, 2011). After running some tests and observing his symptoms, he was also diagnosed with diabetic gastroparesis.

When specifically related to diabetes, it has been seen to occur when the nerves that control the stomach muscles are destroyed over time because of high blood sugar levels. This causes the stomach to empty abnormally, making the person feel full very soon after starting a meal. They may also experience bloating, abdominal pain, severe nausea and vomiting, loss of appetite, heartburn, fluctuations in blood sugar levels, and constipation.

According to healthcare professionals, to manage this condition, patients should eat smaller and more frequent meals low in fat and fiber content so that they are easy to digest and don't put a strain on their gut. Metoclopramide is often used to treat gastroparesis, as it encourages muscles in the stomach to contract and empty the stomach. Even though we are still learning about this disease, with the proper treatment, the symptoms can be managed.

Diverticulitis

Moving our discussion from gastroparesis to diverticulitis, we encounter another problematic and painful disease. Some people develop small sacs on the intestinal lining of the colon, known as diverticula. While diverticula are harmless, sometimes they can get inflamed and cause diverticulitis. Symptoms range from severe abdominal pain and high fever to inflammation and changes in bowel movement.

However, the cause of the disease is unknown. While diverticulosis is common, only 4 percent of those with the disease experience inflammation in the diverticula and develop diverticulitis.

Patients with diverticulitis need to avoid nuts, seeds, and popcorn because these become stuck in the diverticula, causing inflammation to occur and flare-up diverticulitis.

Cancer

Just like cancer can affect any part of the body, it can be fatal to the stomach as well. Cells start producing uncontrollably, lining where the stomach meets the esophagus, which is more common in the US, or in the main part of the stomach, which is usually found in other countries.

These cells can start building up, leading to a tumor that can later spread to other body parts, such as the pancreas and liver, if not removed. In the initial stages, symptoms are not felt physically. However, when they do start showing up, the person must visit a healthcare professional as soon as possible to be tested. Typical symptoms for cancer are loss of appetite, losing a considerable amount of weight without any apparent reason, weakness and constantly feeling tired, nausea and vomiting, black stool, blood in vomit, feeling bloated, and severe stomach pain.

Despite the fact that there is no particular reason why the genetic mutation occurs that causes cancer, certain common factors have been found in people who have this mutation. It's common in males above sixty-five, whose ethnicity originates in East Asia, South or Central America, or Eastern Europe. If someone has a family history of cancer, they are more prone to the occurrence of genetic mutations. Other risk factors include smoking, having a diet with high salt and fats and low in vegetables and fruits, and suffering with other gastric issues on a regular basis.

To lower the risk of getting stomach or colon cancer, eat a low-salt diet and increase vegetable and fruit intake for nutrition. Quitting smoking is highly suggested as well. In cases where cancer does develop, several procedures can be carried out, such as tumor-removing surgery, chemotherapy, radiation, and immunotherapy. Sometimes they are used in combination with each other for the best results. Stomach cancer is indeed curable if it's diagnosed at an early stage. However, typically it's found when a certain amount of time has passed. So, it's best to stay vigilant by employing the methods suggested here to avoid such a circumstance.

Leaky Gut

Leaky gut syndrome is the starting point of most digestive symptoms and diseases. Our gut is semi-permeable; basically, it allows certain things to pass through, like nutrition, and filters out toxins and bad bacteria. Certain people develop an increased permeability, which allows other toxins to pass through as well. There is no medical diagnosis for the condition, and it has no particular cause behind it.

However, it has been found that autoimmune diseases that affect the digestive system cause a leaky gut. In other cases, it was found that certain patients had leaky gut before they were diagnosed with these diseases. It isn't known whether it is the cause of a disease, just another symptom, or if it can be classified as a disease in itself. Regardless, awareness is increasing that leaky gut syndrome is a foundational problem and that it is related to various disease processes.

So, what happens when you have a leaky gut?

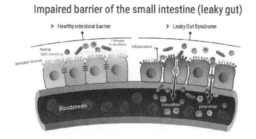

(Image from Alcat-europe – Leaky gut syndrome)

Effects of Leaky Gut

At this point, we have established that an unhappy gut is an unhappy you. The following points highlight how leaky gut syndrome affects the whole digestive system and, in turn, affects your overall health.

- Leaky gut can cause inflammation, which causes your immune system to weaken. It begins to react to every little microbiome in the body, even good ones, which then cause diseases such as irritable bowel disease and arthritis.

- The continual flooding of toxins and bad microbes into the bloodstream causes gut dysbiosis. This is where the bad microbiome increases, creating an imbalance in the gut.

• Additionally, your gut has a lot of bacteria that are responsible for digesting lactose, gluten, and other foods. With a
leaky gut, they all flow out, and the bigger molecules of
food, like proteins, cannot be digested fully, causing food
intolerance.

• The improper in-and-out flow of nutrients through the
bloodstream can also cause nutrient malabsorption, for example, anemia. Moreover, as we've previously seen, gut
health hugely impacts your mental health, as an imbalanced
gut may disrupt the gut-brain axis, leading to the potential
of anxiety and depression.

Gut Check!

The Belly Blueprint Quiz

- How is your daily fruit intake?

1. Fruit? What's that?

2. I eat fruit every few days.

3. I eat fruit daily.

4. I eat loads of fruit daily!

- How many portions of vegetables do you consume daily?

1. I don't eat vegetables at all.

2. I try to eat at least one serving of vegetables a day.

3. I usually eat two servings of vegetables a day.

4. My daily diet is full of tasty vegetables!

- Do you stay hydrated throughout the day?

1. I barely drink any water.

2. I drink 0.5 liters of water a day.

3. I drink about 0.5- 1 liter of water a day.

4. I drink 2 or more liters of water a day.

- How much caffeine do you consume per day? (Includes coffee, tea, caffeinated soft drinks, energy drinks, etc.)

1. I barely drink caffeinated drinks.

2. About 1-2 cups a day.

3. 3 cups a day.

4. 4 or more cups a day.

- How many probiotic foods (yogurt, kefir, etc.) do you eat on a weekly basis?

1. Barely any.

2. 1 serving weekly.

3. About 2-3 servings weekly.

4. More than 3 servings weekly.

- Does your daily diet contain nuts, seeds, or beans?

1. I don't usually have those.

2. About 1-2 servings.

3. 3 servings.

4. More than 4 servings.

- Would you describe your diet as a healthy diet?

1. I eat whatever is convenient, whether it's healthy or not.

2. I try to make my meals as healthy as possible.

3. They are somewhat healthy with a few exceptions at times.

4. It's strictly healthy. I barely eat any extra carbs or fats.

- How many hours do you give yourself after dinner before you go to sleep?

1. I sleep immediately.

2. 1-2 hours.

3. 2-3 hours.

4. 4 or more hours.

- How frequent are your bowel movements?

1. I go once a day, and sometimes not even daily.

2. It's usually once a day.

3. It's twice a day on average.

4. At least three times a day.

- How's your mental state throughout the week?

1. I am fairly unhappy.

2. I am mostly neutral.

3. I feel happy.

- How many hours of sleep do you get every night?

1. I get 5 or less hours of sleep.

2. I sleep 5-7 hours a day.

3. I sleep 7-8 hours a day.

4. I sleep more than 10 hours.

• How often do you exercise for at least thirty minutes to the point that you are short of breath?

1. Sometimes once a week, sometimes I don't at all.

2. About 1-2 times a week.

3. 3-4 times a week.

4. Every. Single. Day. I love working out!

• How often are you bothered by gut discomfort?

1. Less than once a month.

2. About 1 to 3 times a month.

3. Every week.

4. 3 or more times a week.

• Do you take medication or any drugs?

1. Yes.

2. No.

• Do you have health conditions, such as diabetes or blood pressure, running in your family?

1. Yes.

2. No.

I hope you learned something new about yourself in this quiz. You may have discovered that you have a fairly healthy gut, but if, unfortunately, your gut is not healthy and you scored low numbers on this quiz, you need to prioritize yourself and your health more.

What if I told you that what happens in your stomach also directly affects your mood? What if I told you that certain foods can help elevate your mood and aid in removing depression? Incredulous, right? The next chapter will show us how the gut relates to our brain and emotions. It might help you during the times you feel low.

CHAPTER THREE

The Gut–Brain Connection

"Recent studies suggest that in close interactions with its resident microbes, the gut can influence our basic emotions, our pain sensitivity, and our social interactions, and even guide many of our decisions—and not just those about our food preferences and meal sizes."

- Emeran Mayer

The gut-brain connection is remarkable. As communication is bidirectional, it not only serves the digestive system but is also significant in our mental well-being. It's important to understand this connection if you plan to improve your physical and mental health.

Exploring the Gut-Brain Axis

Have you ever been in a situation where you did not logically know what to do, but in the end, you decided to go with your gut? Have you ever experienced butterflies in your stomach when you are nervous about talking to someone you like?

If so, then you already know that our gut and mind are intricately linked with each other. They pass information between each other, discussing all sorts of matters— practical, physical, and emotional—just like best friends do! This connection between your gut and brain is called the gut-brain axis.

In its bidirectional communication, the nerves send information from the gut to the central nervous system and then back from the central nervous system to the gut. The information exchanged can be related to your hunger, food preferences, food intolerances, muscle movements, digestion, metabolism, mood, stress levels, pain sensitivity, cognitive functions, and immunity.

The response that you feel with every exchange of information can vary from fast and potent to gentle and pleasurable. If you get food poisoning and urgently have the need to go to the washroom to empty your bowels, you will experience a fast and potent exchange of information. On the other hand, if you're having a warm cup of hot chocolate on a winter evening, the effect will be gentle and pleasing.

According to clinical evidence, the number of microbes in the gut directly affects the gut-brain axis. Many disorders, such as anxiety, depression, and autism have been shown to have a link with disturbances in the gut. In addition, your diet directly affects your gut, and eventually your cognition. Several studies have proven a link between depression and inflamed cytokines (proteins that help control inflammation in the body). Hence why, in severe depression, patients are given anti-inflammatory drugs, such as COX-2 inhibitors.

In 2017, an experiment was conducted on a sample of forty people with depression. They were asked to take the Beck Depression Inventory test, and their initial responses were recorded. They were then given probiotics (L acidophilus, L casei, and Bifidobacterium bifidum) for eight weeks before taking the Beck Depression Inventory test again. Their responses on the test improved, further proving that having a healthier gut has a significant impact on our mental health (Appleton, 2018).

Through research, we have come to understand that the gut microbiome produces several neurotransmitters that affect mood and cognition. A balanced microbiome community helps keep mood stable and happy, while an imbalance in microbes can cause the inhibition of adequate neurotransmitters. This can lead to an increase in stress levels, and in severe cases, even cause anxiety and depression.

An imbalanced microbiome can also cause internal inflammation, which again lowers the production of required neurotransmitters, leading the person back to an imbalanced microbiome and at an increased risk for lower mood.

Now, we all know the common hormones (neurotransmitters) that determine your happy mood: serotonin and dopamine. Initially, we thought that these hormones were produced in the brain only. However, we now know that many of these are also produced in the gut. For this reason, the gut is also known as the 'second brain.'

Serotonin

Serotonin is a mood-balancing hormone that helps stabilize emotions. Not only does it keep anxiety at bay, but it also helps with digestion, healing wounds, keeping your bowel movements active and functioning normally, and maintaining your bone density. It also activates mucus and fluid secretion inside the digestive system for absorption in the intestine. Serotonin controls nerve receptors as well, which means that it tells you when you feel bloated or are in pain.

The body deals efficiently with serotonin, as any excess is converted to melatonin to help you sleep. Lack of serotonin can be responsible for depression, anxiety, chronic pain, insomnia, and memory issues.

Production and Availability of Serotonin

We now know that 95 percent of serotonin is produced in the gut, while the remaining 5 percent is produced in the brain. Serotonin can only be produced when the gut has the required nutrients to produce it. Nutrients such as vitamin C, vitamin B9, zinc, and omega-3 are essential for the production of serotonin. It really can't be overstated how vital of a role nutrition plays in mental health.

Neurotransmitter Hormones

Dopamine is a neurotransmitter that is necessary for maintaining focus, awareness, productivity, and reproductivity. A lack of dopamine can cause anxiety, an inability to focus, muscle stiffness, and indigestion. 50 percent of dopamine production is carried out in the gut, further reinforcing the importance of the gut-brain axis.

GABA (the major neurotransmitter in the spinal cord that stimulates the production of insulin) is produced in the pancreas, which, if you remember, is also part of the digestive system. GABA reduces stress and anxiety, allowing for relaxation. A lack of it is known to increase the risk of depression, insomnia, and a lack of concentration.

Other neurotransmitter hormones, like norepinephrine (the body's stress response hormone), are also produced in the gut. If your body experiences too much stress and releases a lot of norepinephrine, the excess goes into the gut and weakens the immune system.

Gut-Nourishing Foods

I am often asked, "How can I be happier?" Though there is no one treatment for it, and several mental disorders require you to visit a professional for proper treatment, it is still worth trying a few methods to elevate your mood. In the end, fighting depression requires your own will and steadfastness. The research discussed in this chapter has shown that the gut is very much responsible for our mental health, so the immediate course of action is to improve your routine and remain committed to it, starting with food.

Several of my patients battle with anxiety and mood swings, especially in the presence of various digestive issues. I tell them one thing—your diet determines almost everything, from your health to your mood.

Lisa, aged forty-three, is a mother of two and a high school teacher. For a few months, she was experiencing frequent mood swings and irritability. She felt that sometimes she became passive-aggressive as well with her kids or students. Her work requires her to stay focused and plan lectures accordingly, but she felt she was unable to do her job well because she lacked focus.

She realized that because of her tiring routine, she could not make the time to prepare food herself, which meant eating processed food. After careful discussion, I gave her a simple diet plan that did not require lengthy processes of cooking and suggested she go for a brisk walk for thirty minutes at least four days a week. Five months after her initial check-up, she admitted to feeling much lighter, happier, and focused on her life.

So, what exactly should we be eating to improve our mood?

Foods That Promote Gut Health

As mentioned before, our bodies need prebiotics and probiotics to have a healthier gut. Prebiotics help digestion, control blood sugar levels, and aid in nutrient absorption. Scientists in San Jose University, Boston, Massachusetts, have declared these five foods to be the best sources for prebiotics: garlic, leeks, onions, dandelion greens, and

Jerusalem artichokes. These foods contain about 100-240 milligrams of prebiotics in one gram. On average, an adult human should eat five grams of prebiotics a day.

Nutrient-Rich Foods

Vitamin C is found in citrus fruits like oranges and lemons. It enables the body to process carbohydrates, fats, and proteins. Vitamin C is also an important component in the making of neurotransmitters, such as serotonin, dopamine, and norepinephrine—the hormones that keep depression at a far distance.

In 2018, a study conducted on 139 young men found that those with a good amount of vitamin C in their blood showed the lowest signs of depression (Plevin 2020). For premenstrual depression, vitamin B6 is quite effective. Just like with vitamin C, our bodies require vitamin B6 to produce neurotransmitters.

Additionally, folate—a form of vitamin B9—helps create more cells and DNA, as well as encouraging the production of serotonin, eventually enhancing mood. Another nutrient, magnesium, found in tofu and whole grains, keeps a check on hormonal balance.

And, according to research, it has been found that people with heavy depression often have extremely low zinc levels. Zinc supplements can, therefore, be very therapeutic for people struggling with severe depression.

Last, but not least, since our brain is 60 percent fat, it requires good fats to function well. Omega-3 has been seen to have a significant impact on brain function, reducing the risk of depression in children and adults. The best sources of omega-3 foods are chia seeds, flax seeds, and fish—particularly wild salmon, herring, and sardines. These are low in mercury and high in omega-3. Walnuts also contain a lot of omega-3, as well as helping to lower blood pressure by keeping arteries clean.

To ensure you maintain optimal brain power, eat a good amount of leafy vegetables daily, such as lettuce, spinach, and broccoli. Berries have also been shown to help memory, as proven by researchers at Harvard's Brigham and Women's Hospital (Harvard 2021).

Gut-Friendly Lifestyle Practices for Emotional Balance

Maintaining a healthy gut to achieve good mental health will take time, commitment, and effort. In addition to eating the right foods, including prebiotics, probiotics, and other nutrients, you also need to exercise or do some form of physical workout to activate your gut. You can choose whatever you're comfortable with and enjoy doing, whether walking, jogging, hitting the gym, or even dancing! All you need is 150 minutes a week to sweat. This can help increase the good bacteria in your body by as much as 40 percent.

Besides eating healthily and exercising, try to avoid antibiotics as much as possible. The use of excessive antibiotics can remove the good bacteria as well as the bad from your gut, which can lower your immunity in the long run. Often small issues can be fixed by simple home remedies. If an antibiotic is necessary, take a probiotic at the same time to minimize the assault on your good bacteria.

Gut Health Practices for Enhancing Emotional Resilience and Coping Mechanisms

The most important aspect in keeping your mind healthy is keeping stress low. Although, this is often easier said than done. My immediate response to being stressed used to be binge eating dessert and comfort food. However, I have changed this over the years, and now I try to help other people change their unhealthy reactions to stress, too. You *can* deal with stress using healthy coping mechanisms.

Relaxation Techniques

Start with taking some deep breaths to help your body relax and to regulate your nervous system, calming the fight-or-flight response.

I find the best way to de-stress during a situation is to immediately write about how I'm feeling. I suggest you keep a small journal in your bag, and whenever you feel your emotions are becoming overwhelming, take five minutes and write about it.

Another way to eliminate stressful thoughts about a situation is to think positively, finding the good in a bad situation. Here's an example: you worked really hard for a promotion that was long due, but you didn't get it. This situation can be very demotivating. But it's important to remember that it is not a representation of your skill and hard work. Perhaps you will be rewarded in some other way.

Another idea is to dress up and socialize with your friends; laughing and talking with them can provide you with a good temporary distraction from your stress. They also might have a new perspective on your situation, which could be helpful.

Relaxation or meditation techniques are especially helpful. They can help you pinpoint your emotions and remove the negative energy from within you. One such methodology is the autogenic technique. In this, you use imagery to visualize a peaceful moment or repeat words or phrases that make you feel calm. Then, you focus on your body sensations, being mindful of how each body part reacts, and also noticing your breathing.

The progressive muscle relaxation technique promotes relaxation, too, but utilizes a different method than the autogenic technique. In this, you tense your muscles intentionally and then loosen them to determine the difference between tense muscles because of stress and muscles in a state of relaxation. You start by sitting in a quiet room, devoid of any distractions. You then tense and relax the muscles in your neck for a minute. Next, you work your way down to your shoulders, then the abdomen, your legs, and finally your toes. This technique is especially helpful in making you more aware of your body

.

The third technique, visualization, is similar to the autogenic technique. You sit in a quiet room as relaxed as possible with your shoulders dropped. You may want to close your eyes. Think of a scene that makes you happy and relaxed. For example, sitting by the river where you can hear the gushing sound of the flowing water. Try adding as many elements as you can and want, such as lighting, sunlight, the wind, subjects, and people. Take deep breaths in and out and focus on relaxing your muscles.

Other relaxation techniques include massage, yoga, music therapy, aromatherapy, and hydrotherapy. If you practice these techniques regularly, they can help elevate your mood.

You can also plan a longer time of relaxation—your own self-care week! Here are some ideas for how that could look. Choose to do a thirty-minute simple yoga when you wake up and before breakfast. Yoga helps you stretch your body, strengthen your muscles, and wake up your senses. Then, make an informed choice on the kind of breakfast you want, ensuring it contains enough probiotics and prebiotics. In the evening, go for a thirty-minute brisk walk in nature, and allow yourself to breathe fresh air. If you have a dog, take it out for a run. Your lunch and dinner should include vegetables and fruits, which give you healthy nutrients. Make sure you leave three hours in between your dinner and sleeping time.

On the weekend, take time out for your friends and socialize with them. In addition to that, find some personal 'me' time for yourself, too, doing things that you enjoy. Perhaps you enjoy going out shopping or you like to spread paint on a canvas and create art. Whatever you do, have at least one day to yourself in a week when you can destress yourself. Because the secret to living a happy life is not taking on stress—and a healthy gut!

The next chapter discusses in detail what specific nutrients the organs need to perform best so that you may incorporate them into your daily diet. It will also talk about why it's important to eat mindfully and how it affects your digestion and mood. So, let's read on.

CHAPTER FOUR

Nourishing Your Digestive System

"*The road to good health is paved with good intestines.*"
- Sherry A. Rogers

Welcome to chapter 4, where we're delving into the fascinating world of your digestive system. In the next few pages, we'll uncover the secrets of maintaining a healthy gut.

Here's the plan: this chapter is all about your gut. The goal? To provide you with the essential tools to develop a diet and lifestyle that perfectly aligns with your digestive system. We're not just focusing on what's on your plate; we're exploring a holistic approach to nurturing your gut.

Are you ready to unlock the wonders of nourishment? Let's embark on this journey together as we explore the basic methods for healing your gut through diet and lifestyle choices. Get ready for a personalized and transformative experience!

Balanced Eating for Gut Health

Have you ever contemplated how to maintain a balanced diet for your overall well-being, including the health of your gut? But you didn't know where to start, or perhaps you started and got discouraged with how overwhelming it felt? This section will give you tools and tips to get started and stay on track. Let's navigate through it together.

Sustaining good health and feeling your best heavily relies on maintaining a healthy, balanced diet. While certain groups, such as athletes, might need additional support through protein supplements, most individuals can adequately meet their nutritional needs by embracing a diverse range of foods.

A balanced diet not only fuels your body for effective function but is also instrumental in supporting gut health. Optimal gut function is achieved by consuming a variety of foods, while minimizing the intake of salt, sugars, and saturated fats.

Neglecting a balanced diet can lead to declining nutrient levels, exposing a significant portion of the population to the risk of vitamin deficiencies. Consequences may include problems with digestion, anemia, and skin issues.

Here, we will explore the essentials of a balanced diet, its significance, and practical tips for meeting your nutritional needs daily, with a special focus on how it contributes to maintaining a healthy gut.

Understanding a Balanced Diet

A balanced diet ideally encompasses five food groups, as emphasized by Isabel Maples, a registered dietitian. Each group contributes essential nutrients, such as vitamins, minerals, fiber, and calories. The Dietary Guidelines from the U.S. Department of Agriculture recommend nutrient-dense foods, placing importance on fruits, vegetables, whole grains, dairy, protein foods, and oils (Renton, 2022). These guidelines also stress the importance of limiting added sugars, saturated fats, sodium, and alcohol.

Variety is crucial, particularly concerning the consumption of fruits and vegetables, which also play a key role in promoting a healthy gut. Nutritionist Lamorna Hollingsworth advises aiming for at least five portions a day, regardless of whether they are fresh, frozen, canned, or dried (Renton 2022).

Practical Tips for Maintaining a Balanced Diet Every Day

While a healthy diet includes all necessary nutrients and food groups, maintaining balance is crucial. The plate method, endorsed by Maples, divides your plate into portions for fruits and vegetables, grains, and protein, with dairy on the side. Individualized needs can be assessed using the USDA's MyPlate Plan.

Hollingsworth emphasizes viewing food on a spectrum to avoid labeling it as good or bad. This approach not only promotes overall balance but also fosters gut health, by encouraging the consumption of a variety of foods that nourish the microbiome.

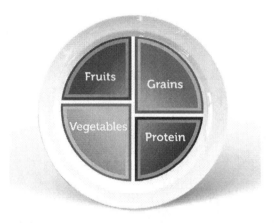

(Image from choosemyplate.gov)

The Power of Probiotics and Prebiotics

As we talked about in Chapter 1, prebiotics are non-digestible fibers that become a feast for the superheroes in your gut: beneficial bacteria. They are the backbone of a healthy gut microbiome, responsible for digestion, immune system harmony, and even mental well-being.

In my journey to better gut health, I found that by incorporating prebiotic-rich foods like chicory root, Jerusalem artichoke, garlic, onions, and bananas into my diet, I witnessed a happier gut, less inflammation, and a newfound energy. It has been truly transformative.

I also started adding more fruits and vegetables to my meals, especially those with complex carbohydrates. These carbs, like fiber and resistant starch, don't get digested by my body. Instead, they become a banquet for bacteria and other microbe rockstars. And when they reach the colon, it's like a celebration. Fermentation occurs, and short-chain fatty acids join the party, bringing a bunch of health perks, such as boosting the immune system, feeling satisfied, and better nutrient absorption. It's like a gut fiesta!

Probiotic-Rich Foods to Add to Your Diet

Have you ever wondered where to find these beneficial bacteria? Well, here's a list of seventeen foods that I personally turn to for their rich probiotic content.

- Kefir: A fermented dairy product similar to yogurt, originating from Russia and Turkey over 3,000 years ago, known for its slightly acidic and tart flavor.

- Sauerkraut: A German favorite, made from fermented cabbage and other probiotic vegetables, it's high in organic acids which support the growth of good bacteria.

- Kombucha: An effervescent fermentation of black tea with primary health benefits including digestive support, increased energy, and liver detoxification.

- Coconut Kefir: Fermented from the juice of young coconuts with kefir grains, it offers a tropical twist along with several strains of beneficial probiotics.

- Natto: A Japanese dish of fermented soybeans containing the powerful probiotic Bacillus subtilis, known for boosting the immune system and supporting cardiovascular health.

- Yogurt: A popular probiotic food made from the milk of cows, goats, or sheep. It does have variations in quality, so opt for organic, grass-fed varieties.

- Kvass: A traditional Eastern European fermented beverage, historically made from rye or barley, now created using probiotic fruits, beets, and other root vegetables.

- Raw Cheese: High in probiotics, including thermophillus, bifidus, bulgaricus, and acidophilus. Choose raw and unpasteurized options for maximum benefits.

- Apple Cider Vinegar: Known for controlling blood pressure, reducing cholesterol, and aiding in weight loss, it can also contribute to your probiotic intake.

- Salted Gherkin Pickles: A lesser-known source of probiotics. Choose smaller, organic producers for the best health benefits.

- Brine-Cured Olives: An excellent probiotic source when brine-cured. Select organic and smaller brands to ensure maximum probiotic content.

- Tempeh: A fermented soybean product from Indonesia, it's versatile and rich in probiotics, suitable for various culinary uses.

- Miso: A traditional Japanese spice created by fermenting soybean, barley, or brown rice with koji, known for its use in miso soup and macrobiotic cooking.

- Traditional Buttermilk: A fermented drink made from the liquid left after churning butter, best when containing live cultures for probiotic benefits.

- Water Kefir: A fizzy, fermented beverage made by adding grains to sugar water, offering a natural, vegan probiotic option with customizable flavors.

- Raw Milk: High in probiotics, particularly when raw and unpasteurized, making it a superior choice compared to pasteurized options.

- Kimchi: The Korean counterpart to sauerkraut. A flavorful mix of fermented vegetables that adds a probiotic boost to your meals.

More Incredible Foods for Gut Health

Now, let's talk about other delicious foods your gut will love. Based on personal experiences and lots of research, here are my recommendations:

- Bananas: Especially the green ones. They're like magic for your gut, and I can vouch for it!

- Artichokes, Broccoli, and Green Peas: Vegetables that are not just good for your taste buds but also pack a punch of fibers and antioxidants for a happy gut.

- Whole Grains: Think oats, brown rice, and whole grain bread. They're like a feast for your gut bacteria fan club.

- Seafood With Omega-3 Fatty Acids: Fish like salmon and mackerel are full of anti-inflammatory powers, promoting gut happiness.

- Fermented Foods: Yogurt, sauerkraut, kimchi, and kombucha are the cool kids with prebiotics that throw the best gut parties.

- Foods with Polyphenols: Dark chocolate, green tea, and red wine—these treats are not just for your taste buds but also a boost for your gut bacteria.

- Almonds: They're not just snacks; they're gut-loving heroes packed with fiber and beneficial fatty acids.

- Ginger: The spicy superhero aiding digestion is a must-have for a happy gut.

- Lean Proteins: Chicken, turkey, eggs, and tofu are not just delicious but also inflammation fighters and gut-lining repair experts. Low-Fructose Fruits: Strawberries, oranges, and blueberries. These fruity delights are gentle on digestion and won't cause a ruckus.

What is the best way to incorporate these into your daily routine? Simple swaps and creative recipes are the key. Substitute soda for kombucha, regular yogurt for the probiotic kind, and experiment with tempeh or sauerkraut for added flavor. Get creative, try new things, and let these probiotic-rich foods enhance your health.

Hydration and its Impact on Digestion

Have you ever thought about the connection between staying hydrated and keeping your gut healthy? We have already talked about how our diet impacts gut health, but let's explore the role that hydration plays in this digestive process.

Water is more than just a drink to quench your thirst; it's a crucial player in various bodily functions, from digestion and nutrient absorption to waste elimination and temperature regulation. Dehydration can actually worsen digestive symptoms, such as constipation and bloating.

So, how does hydration affect gut health? Picture water as the guiding force that helps food move through your digestive tract. It's like the extra push that ensures you have regular bathroom trips. If you're dealing with constipation, increasing your water intake might be the solution.

Here's an interesting fact: Fiber, the superhero nutrient for gut health, needs water as its sidekick. Without enough fluid, too much fiber can lead to discomfort and constipation. Your body might pull extra fluid from the large intestine, making stools hard to pass—a situation you do not want to find yourself in.

Did you know that constipation is the most common cause of bloating? When someone comes to me expressing concerns about bloating, the first thing I check is whether they're dealing with constipation.

Now, let's talk about the practical aspect: How much water do you need? Well, it varies depending on factors like metabolism, environment, and physical activity. As a rough guide, Dietitians of Canada suggest around 2.2 liters (nine cups) for women and 3 liters (twelve cups) for men. Keep in mind that this is a general figure; your unique needs might differ. The more general recommendation is eight cups a day.

Feeling overwhelmed by those water goals? Don't worry! Solid foods contribute about 20 percent of your total water intake. Fruits and veggies, in particular, are packed with water.

For those who find it challenging to drink enough water to take care of the other 80 percent, fear not! There are strategies that can help. Sipping through a straw has been shown to increase water intake. Adding a dash of flavor with mint, citrus, or berries can make hydration more enjoyable. And consider sparkling water since it's a bubbly twist to your plain H2O. To make things easier, carry a water bottle everywhere: in your car, at your desk, you name it.

So, there you have it. A little hydration equals a happy gut. Keep sipping and let your digestive system thank you. Here's to a hydrated and healthy you!

Mindful Eating Practices for Better Digestion

We've all experienced that familiar belly swell after a meal we couldn't resist (the regret of overindulging). It's like a post-feast adventure with buttons popping and cramps setting in. That literal *gut feeling* demands our attention.

Our gut, functioning as the Chief Operating Officer (COO) of our body, holds significant influence. Ever heard of the Enteric Nervous System (ENS)? It's like a hidden brain in our digestive system, impacting our health, mood, and thoughts. Some of us heed its warnings and steer clear of problematic foods, while others persist until resistance builds.

The twist in the tale is this: what you feed your gut matters most. Your food choices dictate your digestive health. The COO sends messages to the brain (the Chief Executive Officer or CEO), triggering various responses. Consume unhealthy foods, and you might find yourself dealing with adult acne, joint pain, or even a canvas of rashes. All because the COO disapproves.

If we're all about becoming healthier, it's time to keep the COO content. A balanced diet, hydration, daily exercise, and quality sleep are the keys to a happy COO. Cut back on culprits like dairy, processed meats, and refined sugars, and witness your gut thriving.

Maintaining a food diary can help you to identify trigger foods—those that leave you feeling low, ones that bring on that unwelcome belly swell, or leave you experiencing other uncomfortable digestive issues. Your gut will thank you for becoming more mindful.

Mindful Eating and its Impact on Digestion

When we embrace mindful eating, we're not just having a meal; we're unlocking a treasure trove of benefits for our overall well-being. By being fully present during our eating experiences, we turbocharge our body's ability to absorb those essential nutrients, creating a healthier digestive haven.

Mindful eating is like a nutrient-absorption superhero. Why? Well, when we're all in on the present moment, our senses kick into high gear and better digestion and absorption follow suit. It's like a nutrient party where we get VIP treatment.

But wait, there's more. Mindful eating isn't just about savoring each bite (though that's pretty awesome); it's a stressbuster, too. Stress messes with nutrient absorption and our gut buddies. However, when we're Zen-like during meals, stress takes a backseat, paving the way for optimal digestion and a thriving gut environment.

A quick tip: Make mindful eating a lifestyle, not just a temporary fling. Despite life's distractions, dedicating yourself to this practice pays off big time. Think about your digestive system doing a happy dance at the improved nutrient absorption as you chew slowly and focus on the sensory delight of eating.

But that's not all, mindful eating is your body's BFF when it comes to hunger signals. No more mindless snacking or overeating. Plus, it's your detective tool to uncover any food triggers or intolerances. Pro tip: Throw in some deep breaths before meals. It's a digestion booster.

Incorporating Mindfulness into Mealtimes

Here are six core tips for mindful eating exercises:

1. Use all your senses: Appreciate flavors, colors, and textures.

2. Eat slowly: Enjoy each bite, focusing on taste and recognizing fullness.

3. No distractions: Put away gadgets and give your meal your full attention.

4. Be thankful: Express gratitude for your food's source.

5. Listen to your body: Pay attention to hunger and fullness cues.

6. Understand emotional eating: Recognize triggers for overeating.

Mindful eating isn't a temporary fix; it's a lifestyle change. Consistency is key for lasting improvements in nutrient absorption and digestive well-being. Take it one bite at a time—little mindful eating adventures for lasting changes in digestive health. If you plan ahead, you can include a variety of healthy options in meals, bringing an interesting variety to your diet.

Mindful eating also encourages other positive changes in everyday life. Because it boosts awareness, encourages mindful choices, and focuses on a satisfying experience, this game-changer for digestive health and your relationship with food will also ripple out in other areas.

Now, let's address the challenges of mindful eating. It takes focus, discipline, and resisting unhealthy temptations. Strategies like planning meals, seeking healthier options, and creating dedicated meal spaces can help. Overcoming distractions and societal pressures means communicating your needs and prioritizing digestive health.

Importance of Chewing Food Properly

Have you ever wondered why our grandparents insisted on chewing food slowly? Well, it's not just an old saying—there's some real wisdom there.

Imagine this: you're digging into a tasty meal, and time is not on your side! We've all been there. But here's the catch: When you scarf down your food like there's a race on, it's like sending a jumbled puzzle to your stomach. Conversely, chewing your food thoroughly is like handing your stomach a set of instructions to solving the puzzle.

I used to be the queen of fast food, always in a hurry. But then, I started getting unwelcome visits from indigestion. I decided to pump the brakes and relish every bite, eliminating the discomfort I felt from speed eating.

When you chew your food well, you're essentially turning it into bite-sized pieces. This not only makes your stomach's job easier but also signals to your body that a feast is on the horizon. Your gut is a fan of mindfulness. It's not just about chewing; it's about being in the moment. When you're conscious of what's going into your mouth, your body responds with a nod of appreciation.

So, the next time you're at the dinner table, put away that phone, take a moment, and chew like it's your first taste. Your gut will send you a thank-you note, and you'll be on your way to a digestive masterpiece.

The Do's and Don'ts of a Gut-Healthy Diet

Ever wondered about inflammation? If you've had a cut, bruise, or throat infection, you've probably felt the signs—redness, swelling, pain, and heat. This is acute inflammation, your body's response to illness or injury, and it usually resolves on its own.

Yet, there's another player: systemic inflammation. It affects the entire body and can last too long. Chronic inflammation is linked to serious diseases like obesity, diabetes, heart disease, and certain cancers. Surprisingly, what you eat can fuel inflammation. Red meat, processed snacks, and sugary drinks all encourage inflammation.

Cooking matters, too. Choose baking, steaming, or a quick stir-fry, since deep frying can stir up trouble. In addition to this, label reading is your weapon against inflammation. Sneaky sugars and trans fats hide in processed foods. If it says, "partially hydrogenated oils," steer clear.

So, what are some anti-inflammatory foods? Think omega-3 fatty acids in fish, vitamin C in fruits and veggies, and polyphenols in coffee, tea, and dark chocolate. And don't forget the gut-friendly squad that we discussed earlier: probiotics and prebiotics in fermented foods and fiber-rich treats.

If you are looking for an MVP diet against inflammation, the Mediterranean diet is your go-to playbook. It's all about omega-3s, vitamin C, polyphenols, and fiber-rich goodness.

Ready to make a change? Start small. Swap out inflammatory culprits for healthier alternatives. Like trading charcuterie for veggie slices with hummus or opting for grilled eggplant instead of a burger. It may seem like a challenge, but these tweaks can turn into habits that kick inflammation to the curb.

Remember, no single food is the hero against inflammation, but crafting a wholesome diet is your superpower. It's not just about reducing risk; it's about transforming your health, one mindful meal at a time.

Strategies to Curb Sugar Cravings and Support Gut Health

Let's talk about overcoming sugar cravings and supporting our gut health. It's a real struggle, and I've been there, grabbing for that sugary fix like it's the solution to everything. But you know what? There are ways to beat those cravings and give our gut some love.

First, let's consider the gut microbiota—those little warriors inside your belly. They play a big role in your cravings and food choices. Personally, I have found that adding more fiber-rich foods to my diet makes a difference. Foods like fruits, veggies, and whole grains have become my allies in this battle.

Now, tackling sugar cravings isn't just about willpower; it's a biochemical challenge. When that sweet tooth kicked in, I started choosing natural sweeteners like honey or maple syrup. These small changes had a significant impact. I also noticed that balancing my meals with protein, healthy fats, and fiber-rich foods helped tone down the intensity of my cravings.

Don't underestimate the power of hydration. I began drinking more water, and surprisingly, my cravings became mere whispers instead of loud demands. Water helped me feel full and satisfied the need to snack on something sweet or salty.

I also embraced mindfulness as a new hobby. When a craving hit, I took a moment to breathe, acknowledged the craving without judgment, and questioned whether I was genuinely hungry or just bored. More often than not, it turned out I was just bored.

Finally, I made sure to have healthy snacks on hand. When the sweet tooth struck, having a stash of nuts, Greek yogurt, or dark chocolate (in moderation) saved me from succumbing to sugary temptations.

To all my fellow sugar warriors, it's not about bidding farewell to sweets forever. It's about finding balance, making mindful choices, and letting your gut be your guide. Trust me, your body will thank you, and those sugar cravings will become a thing of the past.

How to Create and Stick with a New Eating Plan

Healthy eating: it's not just about looking good; it's about feeling good and dodging those nasty diseases. An unhealthy diet? Well, that's the express lane to problems like obesity, heart disease, type 2 diabetes, and even certain cancers.

Now, I get it. Dieting is a beast, but trust me, it's a daily investment in yourself that pays off big time. A healthy diet is only partially about shedding pounds. More importantly, it's about boosting your life expectancy, keeping your immune system in top form, lifting your mood, and ramping up your energy levels so you can conquer your day.

But let's talk about the hurdles. Do you feel like you're stuck in an 'all-or-nothing' loop? One where a tiny slip-up feels like a colossal failure? I've been there, and I want to assure you that it's okay not to be perfect. It's normal to struggle with body image but obsessing over how you look can mess with your healthy eating groove. It's about progress, not perfection.

Stress. Oh boy, stress eating is a thing. I've been there, too. Mindless munching when the world feels heavy. Take a breath; it happens to the best of us. And depression? It's no joke. Poor eating habits can be a sign. If you're battling more than just diet demons and feeling hopeless, chat with your healthcare provider. They've got your back!

So, if any of these hurdles hit close to home, don't rush into a diet plan. Pause and figure out what's holding you back, and then dive in.

Now, let's move on to talking about sticking to your diet plan and actually reaching those goals. I've got a few tips that worked wonders for me:

Keep it Real: Set achievable and realistic goals. Don't go for extreme calorie cuts or expect to lose a ton of weight in a short time. It's not healthy or sustainable.

Start Small: Take it easy at the beginning. Instead of banning entire food groups, try setting small goals like treating yourself once a week.

Going all-in can make it tough to bounce back after the occasional sweet indulgence.

Prep like a Pro: Spend some time each week prepping meals, especially the ones you love. It makes it way easier to choose a home-cooked meal over hitting the drive-through.

Snack Smart: Keep healthy snacks around, whether you're at the office or at home. Frozen grapes or a bit of dark chocolate beat the vending machine any day. Swap out junk for snacks like parmesan crisps or light white cheddar popcorn, which are just as satisfying without the guilt.

Love Your Plan: If your diet is making you miserable, it's not the right one. Find a plan you enjoy like counting macros, where you can still savor your favorite foods in moderation. Talk to your healthcare provider for guidance and maybe some extra tips.

Remember, dieting doesn't have to be a struggle. It's about getting healthier, not just thinner. Slow and steady wins the race. If you need extra support, consider consulting a trained dietitian.

Personalized Approaches to Improving Gut Health

Let's go back to that intricate dance between what we eat, our gut, and our mental well-being. Imagine a world where your diet isn't a generic blueprint but a personalized guide to gut health and mental bliss. Intriguing, right?

I've had my share of battles with digestive issues—bloating, occasional discomfort, and unpredictable tummy troubles. It got me thinking: What if there's more to gut health than a one-size-fits-all approach?

Our guts are as unique as our fingerprints. What works for one may not work for another. It's like trying to force Cinderella's glass slipper onto everyone, a charming idea, but not practical.

Enter personalized nutrition. It considers your quirks, preferences, and even those guilty pleasures that make life delicious. It's about crafting a menu that suits your gut, promoting a symphony of good bacteria while bidding farewell to the mischief-makers.

Now, onto the link between personalized nutrition and mental health. Stress can send your stomach into somersaults. It's a gut feeling (pun intended). Remember, the gut and the brain are in constant communication, influencing moods and mental well-being. Individualized dietary plans bring much-needed support to mental health management. Crafting a daily menu that nourishes your body and shields you against modern stressors empowers you to face life's challenges.

I have also battled stress and mood swings. Aligning my diet with what my body and mind craved lifted the fog. It wasn't an overnight miracle but a gradual transformation, leaving me feeling grounded and emotionally resilient.

So, the takeaway here is simple: your gut is unique, and so should be your approach to nourishing it. Embrace the power of personalized nutrition, not as a trend but as a key to unlocking a happier gut and a more balanced mind. Your body is whispering its needs; all you have to do is listen, one personalized bite at a time.

Create a Gut-Friendly Diet Plan

Now that we've discussed the benefits of tailoring your nutrition to your needs, let's create a meal plan that's kind to your gut. Think of it as a personalized approach to nourishing both your body and mind.

Understand Your Body

- Reflect on how different foods impact you. Take note of any discomfort, bloating, or sensitivities.

- Consider any known food allergies or sensitivities you may have.

Embrace Whole Foods

- Fill your plate with a variety of vegetables and fruits. They're rich in fiber, which is crucial for gut health.

- Choose whole grains such as quinoa, brown rice, and oats for sustained energy and digestive support.

Include Probiotics

- Integrate probiotic-rich foods like yogurt, kefir, sauerkraut, and kimchi. These contribute beneficial bacteria to your gut.

- Explore different fermented foods to find what suits your taste.

Choose Lean Proteins

- Select lean protein sources like chicken, fish, tofu, and legumes. They're gentler on digestion and provide essential amino acids.

- Consider incorporating plant-based protein options for diversity.

Embrace Healthy Fats

- Incorporate sources of healthy fats like avocados, nuts, seeds, and olive oil. They aid in nutrient absorption and support overall well-being.

- Limit saturated and trans fats commonly found in processed foods.

Prioritize Hydration

- Stay adequately hydrated throughout the day. Hydration supports digestion and facilitates nutrient transport.

- Experiment with herbal teas and infused water for added flavor.

Practice Mindful Eating

- Eat slowly and savor each bite. Thoroughly chewing your food aids digestion.

- Consider keeping a food journal to track how your body responds to various meals.

Minimize Processed Foods and Sugars

- Reduce intake of processed foods, which often contain additives that may not be gut-friendly.

- Be mindful of added sugars; opt for natural sweeteners like honey or maple syrup.

Experiment and Listen to Your Body

- Introduce new foods gradually and observe your body's responses.

- Be open to adjusting your meal plan based on what makes you feel the best.

Seek Professional Advice

- If you have specific dietary concerns or health conditions, consult with a registered dietitian or healthcare professional for more personalized guidance.

Remember, this is your journey to a healthier gut. It's about discovering what works uniquely for you. Enjoy your nourishing meals!

CHAPTER FIVE

Lifestyle Choices for Digestive Wellness

Did you know that, on average, 60 to 70 million Americans battle digestive woes? It's time to rewrite your gut's story. For the 73 percent of women facing pre-period digestive blues, and everyone else with a glum tum, this chapter unveils the power of lifestyle choices.

Practical Techniques for Supporting the Gut

While sharing insights on mindful eating is important, it's evident that our bodies require more than that to foster digestive wellness. Let's explore practical techniques that extend beyond our plates, becoming allies in the quest for a healthier gut.

Engage in Purposeful Movement: I've personally found solace in the gentle rhythm of movement. Exercise goes beyond physical sculpting; it's a catalyst for gut health. Simple practices like walking, yoga, or light stretches can stimulate digestion and alleviate bloating.

Harness the Power of Breath: Breathing transcends a reflex. It is also a powerful tool for gut harmony. Mindful breathing techniques, such as diaphragmatic breathing, not only reduce stress but also enhance the parasympathetic nervous system, fostering optimal digestion.

Embrace Stress-Relief Rituals: Stress silently disrupts digestive peace. Through personal exploration, I've uncovered the profound impact of stress-relief practices. From meditation to a warm bath, discover what resonates with you. A calm mind sets the stage for a calm gut.

Practice Abdominal Self-Massage: Visualize a soothing touch that reaches the depths of your gut. Abdominal self-massage, with gentle, circular motions, can alleviate tension, promote blood flow, and awaken the digestive forces within.

Maintain Posture Awareness: Good posture aligns your internal organs, promoting optimal function. Be mindful of how you sit, stand, and move throughout the day. Let your gut benefit from the advantages of proper alignment.

Prioritize Quality Sleep Rituals: Often overlooked, sleep is a cornerstone of well-being. Prioritize a restful night's sleep to allow your body time to repair and rejuvenate. A well-rested gut is better equipped to tackle the challenges of the day.

Embark on this physical journey with me, where each intentional movement becomes a gesture of care for your gut. These practices, combined with mindful dietary choices, form a harmonious symphony that resonates with the rhythm of digestive well-being.

The Connection between Gut Health and Sleep

In my pursuit of a healthier gut, I've uncovered a critical factor that often goes unnoticed: the significance of getting enough quality sleep.

As I delved into the intricate connection between sleep and gut health, it became increasingly clear that the relationship is more profound than I initially thought.

Quality sleep isn't just a luxury; it's a necessity for the well-being of our gut. During the hours we're sleep, our bodies engage in essential repair and rejuvenation processes. This nightly restoration extends its benefits to the gut, contributing to healing, reduced inflammation, and enhanced resilience against digestive issues.

The interdependence between gut health and sleep is fascinating. Not only does sleep nurture the gut, but the state of our gut can also influence the quality of our sleep. Our gut microbes, those tiny inhabitants of our digestive tract, play a crucial role in regulating sleep patterns. The delicate balance of these microbes affects the production of neurotransmitters like serotonin and melatonin, key players in promoting restful sleep.

So, how can we ensure we get enough of this sleep-induced elixir for gut healing? Here are some personal insights I've gathered along the way:

Establish a Consistent Sleep Routine: Like our digestive system, our sleep cycle thrives on regularity. Set a consistent bedtime and wake-up time to sync with your body's internal clock.

Create a Relaxing Bedtime Ritual: Wind down before bed with calming activities. Whether it's reading a book, gentle stretches, or a warm bath, these rituals signal to your body that it's time to prepare for rest.

Mind Your Gut-Friendly Diet: Your daytime eating habits can impact your sleep. Opt for gut-friendly foods, such as fiber-rich fruits and vegetables, and consider a balanced evening meal to avoid disrupting your digestive system during the night.

Limit Stimulants before Bed: Caffeine and electronic devices can interfere with both gut health and sleep. Minimize these stimulants in the hours leading up to your bedtime routine.

Prioritizing sufficient sleep that is high in quality has become a cornerstone of my journey toward optimal gut health. In the quiet moments of the night, the magic unfolds, weaving together the threads of gut healing and peaceful slumber.

Exercise and Digestion

Exercise is a dynamic force that influences the gut in multifaceted ways. One notable benefit is the promotion of a diverse and flourishing gut microbiome. Engaging in regular workouts increases the abundance and variety of beneficial microbes, contributing to a more resilient and balanced gut ecosystem.

Exercise also plays a pivotal role in enhancing gut motility—the rhythmic contraction and relaxation of the intestinal muscles that drive food movement. This not only aids digestion but also helps prevent issues like constipation, fostering a smoother and more efficient gut.

The impact of exercise on emotional resilience adds another layer to this narrative. In my own journey of embracing physical activity, I found that it led to a positive shift in my mood and stress levels. Regular exercise has a profound impact on the release of neurotransmitters like endorphins and serotonin, known as the feel-good chemicals. These neurotransmitters not only uplift mood but also contribute to a more balanced and resilient emotional state.

As we recently delved into, in the realm of gut health, the gut-brain axis takes center stage. This bidirectional communication highway connects the gut and the brain, influencing both digestive processes and emotional well-being. Exercise, it turns out, is a powerful conductor on this axis, fostering a harmonious interplay between the gut and the brain.

As I integrated exercise into my routine, it became more than just a physical practice; it became a sanctuary for emotional release and resilience. The meditative rhythm of a run, the empowering feeling of lifting weights, or the grounding nature of yoga all became avenues for promoting gut health and cultivating emotional strength.

So, how can you embark on this journey of integrating exercise into your life for the betterment of gut health and emotional resilience? Here are a few personal insights:

Find Joy in Movement: Discover physical activities that bring you joy. Whether it's dancing, hiking, or practicing martial arts, choose activities that resonate with you.

Consistency Matters: Aim for regularity rather than intensity. Consistent, moderate exercise has been shown to yield long-term benefits for both gut health and emotional well-being.

Listen to Your Body: Pay attention to how your body responds to different forms of exercise. This mindful approach helps tailor your routine to suit your unique needs.

Combine Aerobic and Strength Training: Incorporating a mix of aerobic exercises and strength training will benefit cardiovascular health and muscle strength while contributing to a well-rounded impact on gut health.

Now that we've looked at how to incorporate exercise into your routine, let's look at the different types of exercise that can be incorporated and the benefits they bring to gut health.

Aerobic Exercise (e.g., Brisk Walking, Jogging, Cycling)

Duration: Aim for at least 30 minutes of moderate-intensity aerobic exercise most days of the week.

Benefits: Aerobic activities stimulate the digestive system, promoting regular bowel movements and reducing the risk of constipation.

Yoga

Duration: A 20- to 30-minute yoga session several times a week will help you feel its benefits the most.

Benefits: Yoga poses, especially those focusing on twisting and bending, can massage the abdominal organs, improving digestion and reducing bloating.

Strength Training (e.g., Weightlifting, Resistance Exercises)

Duration: Include strength training exercises two to three times a week, targeting major muscle groups.

Benefits: Building muscle mass can boost metabolism and promote overall bodily function, including digestion.

Walking after Meals

Duration: A 10- to 15-minute walk after meals can be effective.

Benefits: Walking aids in the movement of food through the digestive tract, helping to prevent indigestion and promoting better nutrient absorption.

High-Intensity Interval Training (HIIT)

Duration: Short, intense bursts of exercise (15 to 30 minutes) interspersed with rest.

Benefits: HIIT can improve overall fitness and may enhance metabolism, contributing to better digestion.

It's important to choose activities that you enjoy and can maintain consistently. Always consult with a healthcare professional or fitness expert before starting a new exercise regimen, especially if you have any pre-existing health conditions.

Tailoring your exercise routine to your preferences and physical condition will make it more sustainable, ensuring that movement becomes a positive and regular contributor to your digestive well-being.

Real Life Changes from Exercise

Eva's Journey to Improved Digestion through Running

Eva had been grappling with sluggish digestion and frequent indigestion for years. Tired of the cycle of discomfort, she decided to make running a regular part of her routine. As she started incorporating running into her life, Eva not only experienced improvements in her cardiovascular health but also noticed a significant positive change in her digestive well-being. The rhythmic motion of running seemed to invigorate her digestive system, leading to more regular bowel movements and a visible reduction in bloating.

Jake's Digestive Miracle with HIIT Workouts

Jake, a fitness enthusiast, always enjoyed high-intensity workouts. Little did he know that these intense sessions would bring unexpected relief to his digestive problems. Dealing with occasional constipation and discomfort, Jake found that his commitment to vigorous exercise became a game-changer. The increased blood flow and elevated heart rate seemed to enhance gut motility (the ability of organisms and fluid to move or get around), providing a natural solution to his digestive woes. Jake's experience highlights how intense workouts can positively impact both physical fitness and digestive comfort.

Yoga and Gut Harmony

Before we move on from exercise, it's important to spend a little more time focusing on yoga. Gut harmony and yoga are closely linked, in that they both play vital roles in overall well-being. See the following for various ways the gut and the mind are connected:

Stress Reduction

Yoga is recognized for its stress-reducing benefits, which is important for the gut because stress is known to impact the gut negatively through issues like inflammation and changes in gut microbiota. Practices such as deep breathing and meditation in yoga activate the relaxation response, reducing stress levels and contributing to a healthier gut environment.

Mind-Body Connection

The gut-brain axis is influenced by emotional and psychological factors. Yoga emphasizes the mind-body connection, encouraging practitioners to be present and mindful during their practice.

Physical Movement

Yoga involves physical postures and movements that stimulate the digestive organs. Twisting poses, for instance, can massage the digestive tract and improve digestion. This helps regulate bowel movements and prevent constipation, promoting a healthier gut.

Breath Control (Pranayama)

The breath control exercises practiced in yoga directly impact the autonomic nervous system, which influences the balance between the sympathetic and parasympathetic branches. Deep diaphragmatic breathing in yoga activates the parasympathetic nervous system, enhancing digestion and nutrient absorption by promoting a state of relaxation.

Holistic Wellness

Holistic wellness is crucial for maintaining a healthy gut. Yoga promotes this by addressing mental, emotional, and physical well-being.

While yoga can contribute to gut harmony, individual responses may vary. Adopting a comprehensive approach to health, including a balanced diet, regular exercise, and proper hydration alongside yoga practices, can maximize benefits for gut health. Always consult healthcare professionals for personalized advice, especially if you have specific gut-related concerns or conditions (Jain, 2023).

Stories of Gut-Health Victories from Yoga

Eleana's Stress Relief

Eleana, a twenty-eight-year-old professional juggling a demanding job, struggled with persistent digestive issues. Seeking relief, she turned to yoga. Consistent practice, focusing on stress-reducing poses and mindful breathing, brought a notable improvement in her digestion. The mind-body connection fostered by yoga became a key element in Eleana's overall well-being.

Tom's IBS Management

Tom, a thirty-eight-year-old with irritable bowel syndrome (IBS), found solace in yoga. Initially hesitant, he began with beginner-friendly classes emphasizing controlled breathing and gentle movements. As he maintained a regular practice, Tom experienced reduced stress levels and a significant decrease in the frequency and severity of his digestive issues. Yoga became a vital part of his daily routine, providing both serenity and digestive comfort.

Yoga Poses That Aid Digestion and Reduce Stress

I've discovered a set of yoga poses that have been beneficial for improving digestion and alleviating specific digestive issues. Here's a brief guide to some of my favorite poses:

- *Seated Side Bend (Parsva Sukhasana):* A beginner-friendly move that stretches obliques, belly muscles, and the upper and lower back, providing relief from bloating and gas.

- *Seated Twist (Ardha Matsyendrasana):* This twisting pose promotes bowel regularity, aiding the small and large intestines. It's effective in reducing bloating and enhancing digestion.

- *Supine Spinal Twist (Supta Matsyendrasana):* Ideal for stretching the lower back and increasing spinal mobility, believed to alleviate constipation, bloating, and support general digestion.

- *Knees to Chest (Apanasana):* A gentle movement that relaxes and relieves lower back strain, with claims of massaging the large intestine to promote bowel movements.

- *Cat-Cow (Marjaryasana-Bitilasana):* Transitioning between cat pose and cow pose, these stretches improve circulation and gently massage organs to promote gut peristalsis.

- *Cobra Pose (Bhujangasana):* This pose mimics a cobra's upright position, stretches belly muscles, improves posture, and is believed to support overall digestion (Sullivan, 2021).

Incorporating these poses into my routine has been a game-changer for my digestive well-being. Remember to practice each pose mindfully, focusing on deep breaths and maintaining proper form.

Smoking and Your Gut

Smoking has detrimental effects on the digestive system, increasing the chances of heartburn, peptic ulcers, and complications in their treatment. It also raises the risk of Crohn's disease, gallstones, and exacerbates liver disease and pancreatitis. Furthermore, there is a correlation between smoking and cancers in digestive organs, including the head, neck, stomach, pancreas, and colon.

All in all, quitting smoking is crucial to reducing the risk of various digestive disorders, cancers, and associated health complications. Seeking professional assistance can be beneficial in the journey of quitting to improve overall digestive health.

Alcohol Consumption

Excessive alcohol consumption can have a range of negative impacts on gut health, extending beyond common issues, such as hangovers. While moderate drinking (up to one drink a day for women and two drinks a day for men) is generally considered safe, surpassing these limits can lead to potential problems. These include:

Acid Reflux: Alcohol relaxes the lower esophageal sphincter, causing acid reflux or heartburn. Persistent acid reflux may lead to more severe conditions like Barrett's esophagus or esophageal cancer.

Diarrhea: Alcohol disrupts the balance of gut bacteria, promoting inflammation and leading to a leaky gut. This condition allows toxins to enter the bloodstream, contributing to diarrhea.

Gastritis: Excessive alcohol disrupts mucus production in the stomach, causing inflammation known as gastritis. Repeated episodes can lead to ulcers, anemia, or stomach cancer.

Bloating: Alcohol affects sugar digestion and alters the balance of gut bacteria, leading to bloating. Beer is more commonly associated with this issue compared to wine or spirits.

Liver Damage: Heavy alcohol use can result in alcoholic fatty liver disease, leading to liver failure, cancer, or cirrhosis over time. Early detection through routine bloodwork allows for reversibility with lifestyle changes.

Pancreatic Damage: Alcohol can damage the pancreas, causing in-flammation (pancreatitis). This condition can be life-threatening, especially for heavy drinkers and smokers, increasing the risk of organ failure and long-term complications, such as diabetes and pancreatic cancer.

Treatment for alcohol-induced pancreatitis can be administered in various ways, including IV fluids, electrolyte replacement, tube feeding, and counseling for alcohol cessation. Severe cases may necessitate surgery and involve a lengthy recovery, with potential long-term complications. It is crucial to be aware of these risks and seek medical advice for moderation or cessation of alcohol consumption.

The Impact of Antibiotics on Gut Flora

Antibiotics play a crucial role in treating bacterial infections but can disrupt the delicate balance of gut flora. These medications, designed to target specific bacteria, often affect both harmful and beneficial microbes in the gastrointestinal tract, leading to a potential reduction in microbial diversity. This disturbance may result in various digestive issues and an increased vulnerability to infections.

Prolonged antibiotic use could also have lasting effects on gut flora, potentially contributing to conditions like irritable bowel syndrome (IBS) or inflammatory bowel disease (IBD).

To mitigate these effects, it is important to use antibiotics judiciously and consider counter-measures, such as incorporating pro-biotics or prebiotics post-treatment, to support the restoration of a healthy gut microbiome.

Food Intolerances and Sensitivities

Recognizing and addressing food intolerances can pose challenges, yet it is crucial for enhancing one's health. Distinguishing itself from allergies, food intolerance doesn't involve the immune system but arises from difficulties in digesting specific foods, like lactose.

Causes include insufficient digestive enzymes, potential nutritional deficiencies, prolonged illnesses, or sensitivities to certain foods like gluten. Precise diagnosis requires assessment by specialists, such as allergists or dietitians, and typically involves blood and skin tests. Once identified, managing food intolerances involves steering clear of problematic foods, using digestive enzyme supplements, and monitoring nutritional intake.

Adopting lifestyle changes, including stress reduction, regular exercise, and mindful eating, can alleviate symptoms and promote overall well-being. Taking a proactive stance and seeking professional guidance when necessary are pivotal steps in navigating food intolerances.

Common Symptoms of Food Intolerances

Food intolerances can lead to various uncomfortable symptoms, such as bloating, gas, and abdominal pain. These symptoms may resemble those of conditions like inflammatory bowel disease and celiac disease.

The manifestations of food intolerance can differ among individuals and may be influenced by factors like the quantity and type of food consumed. Digestive issues are common, but skin and joint symptoms can also arise. Symptoms typically emerge within 30 minutes to 48 hours after consuming the problematic food.

Common intolerances, such as lactose intolerance, affect a significant portion of the global population. Naturally occurring chemicals in food, such as glutamate, salicylates, and amines, contribute to intolerance.

Beyond gastrointestinal symptoms, other effects may include nausea, vomiting, acid reflux, migraines, fatigue, and irritability, which highlights the diverse impact of food intolerance on overall well-being.

Elimination Diets for Identifying Food Intolerances and Sensitivities

An elimination diet can be effective in addressing inflammation and gastrointestinal issues by temporarily removing specific foods. There are various approaches to this diet, such as Whole30, autoimmune protocol, low-FODMAP, and Specific Carbohydrate Diet, among others, each with its own set of guidelines. Some diets also recommend reducing sugar, caffeine, and alcohol intake.

During the elimination phase, which typically lasts one to three months, strict adherence is crucial to accurately assess improvements in symptoms. It's important to note that inflammatory reactions to certain foods may persist for up to two weeks after ingestion. Therefore, maintaining strict compliance during this phase is essential for optimal results.

Equally important is the reintroduction phase, where each eliminated food is systematically reintroduced, following a protocol of incremental intake over two to three days. This is proceeded by an observation phase for three to four days. Keeping a food and symptom diary helps track unexpected benefits or adverse reactions.

Symptoms to monitor during reintroduction include skin changes, mood swings, headaches, sleep disturbances, nasal congestion, fluid retention, joint or muscle pain, fatigue, and gastrointestinal issues. The goal is to gather comprehensive knowledge about how different foods impact individual well-being, enabling informed decisions on whether to avoid certain foods or consume them in moderation.

After completing the elimination diet, it is advisable to adhere to good nutrition principles by incorporating a variety of whole-plant foods, while at the same time limiting added-sugar and processed foods. This ensures a balanced and healthy dietary approach moving forward.

How to Manage Food Intolerances in Daily Life

Identify Triggers: Work with a professional to pinpoint trigger foods through tests or an elimination diet.

Educate Yourself: Learn about alternative ingredients and read labels to avoid hidden intolerant-inducing components.

Meal Planning: Plan meals, opting for homemade options to control ingredients.

Communication: Communicate intolerance to others, especially when dining out.

Choose Whole Foods: Prioritize unprocessed options, such as fresh fruits, vegetables, lean proteins, and whole grains.

Experiment with Cooking: Try different cooking methods, and use herbs and spices for flavor without triggering intolerances.

Read Labels: Thoroughly read food labels to identify potential allergens or intolerant-inducing ingredients.

Carry Safe Snacks: Keep safe snacks on hand for situations with limited food options.

Stay Informed: Stay updated on new products and changes in ingredient formulations.

Consult Professionals: Regularly consult with healthcare professionals or dietitians to ensure nutritional needs are met.

Gut Reset

A gut reset involves making intentional dietary and lifestyle changes to promote a healthier gut microbiome. This typically includes eliminating potential irritants, introducing gut-friendly foods, incorporating probiotics, staying hydrated, and managing stress. The duration varies, and consulting healthcare professionals for personalized guidance is advisable. The goal is to support digestion, address gut-related issues, and enhance overall well-being.

Success Stories

Paul's Achievements

Paul successfully lowered his blood pressure, increased focus, and achieved weight loss through a gut reset. Despite facing a demanding job and a hectic lifestyle, the reset reduced his blood pressure and left him feeling more energized and significantly sharper. Additionally, he experienced significant weight loss.

Megan's Progress

Megan found relief beyond prescribed medications for her chronic stomach conditions through a gut reset. Dealing with Barrett's, esophagitis, and reflux disease, along with insomnia, aches, and low energy, Megan decided to try the cleanse based on a friend's suggestion. To her surprise, the reset alleviated her stomach issues more effectively than the prescribed medication and improved her sleep and overall well-being.

The Benefits and Limitations of a Gut Reset

Benefits of a Gut Reset:

Improved Digestive Health: A gut reset can help alleviate digestive issues, such as bloating, gas, and irregular bowel movements. It allows the digestive system to recalibrate and function more efficiently.

Balanced Gut Microbiome: Resetting the gut often involves introducing probiotics and prebiotics, fostering a balanced and diverse gut microbiome. This can positively impact overall health, including immune function and mental well-being.

Increased Nutrient Absorption: A healthier gut environment enhances the absorption of nutrients from food, ensuring that the body receives the necessary vitamins and minerals for optimal functioning.

Weight Management: Some individuals experience weight loss as a result of a gut reset. This may be attributed to improved digestion, reduced inflammation, and better metabolism.

Enhanced Energy Levels: By promoting efficient digestion and nutrient absorption, a gut reset can lead to increased energy levels. Individuals often report feeling more vibrant and alert.

Improved Mental Health: Because of the link between the gut and mental health, a gut reset may contribute to improved mood and cognitive function, although individual responses vary.

Limitations of a Gut Reset:

Individual Variability: Responses to a gut reset can vary significantly among individuals. What works well for one person may not yield the same results for another, as each person's microbiome and health conditions are unique.

Temporary Effects: The benefits of a gut reset may be temporary if underlying lifestyle factors, such as poor dietary choices or high stress levels, are not addressed in the long term. Maintenance of a healthy gut requires ongoing lifestyle choices.

Potential Discomfort: Some individuals may experience discomfort or mild side effects during the initial phases of a gut reset. This can include changes in bowel habits, bloating, or gas. These symptoms are often transient but are worth mentioning.

Consultation Requirement: Before undertaking a gut reset, individuals with pre-existing health conditions should consult with healthcare professionals. This is crucial to ensure that the reset aligns with their specific health needs and doesn't pose any risks.

A gut reset can offer various benefits, particularly in improving digestive health and promoting overall well-being. However, it is essential to approach it with an understanding of individual variability and the need for sustained healthy habits.

Step-by-Step Guide to a Safe Gut Reset

1. Consult a Professional:
- Seek advice from a healthcare professional before making any significant changes

2. Gradual Diet Changes:
- Increase fiber intake with fruits, vegetables, and whole grains.

  - Include an assortment of fruits, vegetables, whole grains, and legumes in your meals.

  - Fiber promotes digestive regularity and nurtures beneficial gut bacteria.

- Include probiotic-rich foods or supplements.

  - Integrate probiotic-rich foods like yogurt, kefir, sauerkraut, or kimchi into your diet.

  - If necessary, consider a high-quality probiotic supplement.

- Stay hydrated with plenty of water.

  - Begin your day with a glass of water to initiate hydration.

  - Strive to consume at least eight glasses of water throughout the day.

- Include soothing herbal teas, like peppermint or ginger, known for aiding digestion.

3. Elimination Phase:

- Reduce processed and sugary foods.

- Opt for whole, unprocessed foods to foster a diverse microbiome.

- Consider an elimination diet under professional guidance.

4. Mindful Eating:

- Chew thoroughly.

- Establish regular mealtimes.

- Eat without distractions.

5. Stress Management:

- Engage in regular exercise.

- Practice mindfulness activities like meditation or yoga.

6. Sleep Health:

- Maintain a consistent sleep schedule.

- Establish a relaxing bedtime routine.

7. Reintroduction:

- After a few weeks, gradually reintroduce eliminated foods and observe how your body reacts.

- Gradually reintroduce eliminated foods one at a time.

- Monitor your body's response.

8. Long-Term Maintenance:

- Adopt a balanced, varied diet for sustained gut health.

- Set consistent mealtimes to uphold a regular eating schedule.

- Incorporate healthy snacks, if necessary, to prevent extended periods without food.

- Regularly assess and adjust your lifestyle.

- Diminish the consumption of caffeinated beverages and alcohol, recognizing their potential impact on gut health.

9. Regular Check-ins:
- Schedule follow-ups with a healthcare professional.

- Discuss progress and make adjustments as needed

Remember, personalization and professional guidance are essential for a safe and effective gut reset. Always pay attention to your body's signals and make adjustments based on your individual needs and preferences.

The Role of Healthcare Professionals in Guiding a Gut Reset

Take care when choosing a healthcare professional because they play a pivotal role in guiding a safe and effective gut reset. Through individualized assessments, they will tailor the reset plan to your unique health profile, identifying underlying issues and any potential risks. Then, armed with evidence-based practices, they will offer recommendations for gradual dietary changes, help you monitor your progress, and make any necessary adjustments.

Collaboration with a specialist will ensure you receive comprehensive care that prioritizes the individual's well-being. The specialist will also educate and empower you, fostering sustainable habits for long-term gut health beyond the reset period.

Revitalize 360

Boost Immunity, Ignite Wellbeing, & Transform Your Gut Health for a Harmonious, Radiant You!

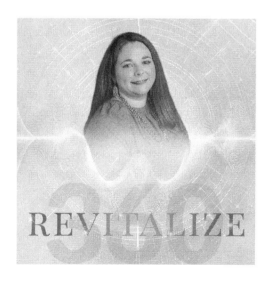

Dr. Ashley's 90-day Gut Reset Program

If you're ready to supercharge your gut health with personalized guidance, my Group Gut Healing Program is designed for you. Join a community of like-minded individuals on a transformative journey to optimal gut wellness.

- Decrease symptoms of bloating, gas, constipation, diarrhea

- Improve nutrient absorption to support body function

- Reduce fatigue and improve energy levels to increase activity and engagement

- Establish more mental clarity

- Boost immune function

- Improve skin blemishes

- Reduce chronic inflammation

Program Includes:
- Lab diagnostics

- 1:1 lab review

- 30-day detox

- 90-day replenishment

- Complete PDF guide

- Unlimited group access: No expiration, Continued support, Q & A calls, Topic discussions

Check it out HERE! https://ashleysullivanonline.com/products -and-services/revitalize-360-product-page

CHAPTER SIX

Healing Herbs and Remedies

"All those spices and herbs in your spice rack can do more than provide calorie-free, natural flavorings to enhance and make food delicious. They're also an incredible source of antioxidants and help rev up your metabolism and improve your health at the same time." - Suzanne Somers

Chapter 6 is all about simple and natural ways to keep your stomach healthy with herbs and remedies that come from nature to support your gut. The goal is to help you learn about these natural options, so that you feel confident using them to improve your own gut health.

Herbal Allies for the Gut

Numerous herbs are recognized for their potential advantages in promoting a healthy digestive system. These herbs are believed to contribute to the alleviation of digestive problems, reduction of inflammation, and the support of a thriving gut microbiome. The following herbs are commonly associated with promoting gut health:

Peppermint (Mentha piperita)

Benefits: Eases symptoms of irritable bowel syndrome (IBS), including abdominal pain and bloating. It possesses anti-inflammatory and antispasmodic properties.

Ginger (Zingiber officinale)

Benefits: Facilitates digestion, alleviates nausea, and may assist with indigestion. Ginger is known for its anti-inflammatory and antioxidant properties.

Turmeric (Curcuma longa)

Benefits: Contains curcumin, which exhibits anti-inflammatory and antioxidant properties. It may aid in reducing symptoms associated with inflammatory bowel diseases (IBD).

Chamomile (Matricaria chamomilla)

Benefits: Soothes the digestive tract, diminishes indigestion, and may alleviate symptoms of IBS. Chamomile has anti-inflammatory and calming effects.

Fennel (Foeniculum vulgare)

Benefits: Alleviates bloating, gas, and indigestion. Fennel seeds have historical use as a digestive aid.

Licorice (Glycyrrhiza glabra)

Benefits: Assists in soothing the stomach lining and may be utilized to address symptoms of heartburn and ulcers. It exhibits anti-inflammatory properties.

Aloe Vera (Aloe barbadensis miller)

Benefits: Aloe vera gel may aid in managing digestive issues like constipation and irritable bowel syndrome. It possesses anti-inflammatory and soothing properties.

Dandelion (Taraxacum officinale)

Benefits: Supports liver health, indirectly benefiting digestion. Dandelion root is occasionally used as a mild laxative and digestive aid.

Slippery Elm (Ulmus rubra)

Benefits: Soothes the digestive tract and may be helpful for conditions such as gastritis and acid reflux. It forms a protective layer in the digestive tract.

Marshmallow Root (Althaea officinalis)

Benefits: Contains mucilage, offering soothing and protective effects on the digestive tract. It may be employed for conditions like gastritis and heartburn.

Lemon Balm (Melissa officinalis)

Benefits: Exhibits mild calming effects and may assist with indigestion and gas. Lemon balm promotes relaxation, which is advantageous for digestion.

Cinnamon (Cinnamomum verum)

Benefits: May contribute to regulating blood sugar levels and improving insulin sensitivity, indirectly benefiting gut health.

Coriander (Coriandrum sativum)

Benefits: Aids digestion, reduces gas, and may alleviate symptoms of irritable bowel syndrome (IBS). Coriander has anti-inflammatory properties.

Mint (Mentha spp.)

Benefits: Eases indigestion, reduces gas, and may provide relief from symptoms of IBS. Mint also has a calming effect on the digestive tract.

Rosemary (Rosmarinus officinalis)

Benefits: Supports digestion, reduces bloating, and has antimicrobial properties that may contribute to a healthy gut environment.

Oregano (Origanum vulgare)

Benefits: Possesses antimicrobial and anti-inflammatory properties, which can support a balanced gut microbiome and alleviate digestive discomfort.

Holy Basil (Ocimum sanctum)

Benefits: Known for its adaptogenic properties, holy basil may help the body manage stress, which can have a positive impact on digestive health.

Thyme (Thymus vulgaris)

Benefits: Supports digestion, reduces inflammation, and has antimicrobial properties that may aid in maintaining a healthy balance of gut bacteria.

Rose Hip (Rosa canina)

Benefits: Rich in antioxidants, rose hip may contribute to reducing inflammation in the digestive system and support overall gut health.

Nettle (Urtica dioica)

Benefits: Supports the liver and may indirectly benefit digestion. Nettle tea is often used as a gentle digestive tonic.

Cumin (Cuminum cyminum)

Benefits: Aids digestion, reduces bloating, and may help alleviate symptoms of indigestion. Cumin also has antimicrobial properties.

Astragalus (Astragalus membranaceus)

Benefits: Known for its immune-boosting properties, astragalus may contribute to overall gut health by supporting the body's defenses.

Catnip (Nepeta cataria)

Benefits: Has calming effects on the digestive system, reducing indigestion and bloating. Catnip tea is commonly used for digestive comfort (*Explore The 12 Best Herbs for Digestion*, 2022).

Vitamins

Vitamins, minerals, and antioxidants play critical roles in supporting optimal gut function. Listed within this section are key nutrients that are particularly important for promoting gut health. Recommended dosages and usage guidelines are also included.

- Vitamin D:

  - Role: Essential for regulating the immune system, so it has the potential to reduce gut inflammation.

  - Additional Benefits: Facilitates calcium absorption, contributing to the maintenance of a healthy gut lining.

  - Recommended Daily Allowance (RDA): It is advisable to adhere to the daily intake levels recommended by health authorities to support overall health.

- Vitamin C:

  - Role: Functions as an antioxidant, playing a pivotal role in supporting the immune system.

  - Additional Benefits: May help mitigate oxidative stress within the gut.

  - RDA: Meeting the recommended daily intake of vitamin C is crucial for its various health-promoting effects.

- Vitamin A:

  - Role: Critical for preserving the integrity of the gut lining.

  - Additional Benefits: Supports the health of mucous membranes within the digestive system.

  - RDA: Adhering to the recommended daily intake of

Vitamin A is important for sustaining gut health and overall well-being.

- Vitamin E:

    ○ Role: Functions as an antioxidant, providing protection against oxidative damage to the gut lining.

    ○ RDA: Ensuring an adequate intake of Vitamin E is essential in harnessing its protective effects on the digestive system.

Understanding the significance of these nutrients in the context of digestive health underscores the importance of maintaining a balanced and varied diet. Including a diverse range of foods rich in these vitamins contributes to the upkeep of a healthy gut and overall well-being.

Minerals
- Calcium:

    ○ Role: Essential for muscle function within the digestive tract.

    ○ Additional Benefits: Maintains the tight junctions of the gut lining, contributing to the overall structural integrity of the digestive system.

- Magnesium:

    ○ Role: Supports muscle contractions in the digestive system.

    ○ Additional Benefits: Regulates bowel movements, aiding in the overall coordination and efficiency of the digestive process.

- Zinc:

  - Role: Contributes to maintaining the integrity of the gut lining.

  - Additional Benefits: Supports immune function, playing a vital role in the body's defense mechanisms related to digestive health.

- Iron:

  - Role: Essential for the formation of hemoglobin, which transports oxygen to cells, including those in the digestive tract.

  - Additional Benefits: Supports overall energy metabolism, crucial for the efficient functioning of digestive organs.

- Potassium:

  - Role: Facilitates proper muscle contractions, including those involved in digestion.

  - Additional Benefits: Maintains fluid balance, aiding in the prevention of dehydration, which is important for healthy digestion.

- Selenium:

  - Role: Functions as an antioxidant, protecting cells in the digestive system from oxidative damage.

- ○ Additional Benefits: Supports the immune system and may contribute to the prevention of inflammation in the digestive tract.

- Copper:

  - ○ Role: Plays a role in the formation of connective tissue, which is essential for the structural integrity of the digestive organs.

  - ○ Additional Benefits: Contributes to the absorption and utilization of iron, supporting overall digestive function.

- Manganese:

  - ○ Role: Participates in the metabolism of amino acids and carbohydrates, supporting the energy needs of digestive tissues.

  - ○ Additional Benefits: Acts as an antioxidant, helping to protect cells in the digestive system from oxidative stress.

Incorporating a diverse range of nutrient-rich foods into your diet ensures an adequate intake of these minerals, promoting digestive health and overall well-being.

Antioxidants

Antioxidants play a crucial role in promoting digestive health by counteracting oxidative stress and inflammation. Here are several antioxidants, each with unique contributions to safeguarding the gut:

- **Glutathione:**

- A potent antioxidant known for its ability to protect the gut lining from oxidative stress and inflammation.

- Glutathione serves as a key defender against harmful free radicals, thereby supporting the overall well-being of the digestive system.

- **Quercetin:**

  - Found in foods like apples, onions, and berries, quercetin is an antioxidant with potential anti-inflammatory properties.

  - Its presence in various fruits and vegetables highlights its role in mitigating inflammation within the gut, contributing to digestive wellness.

- **Polyphenols:**

  - These antioxidants, abundant in foods like green tea, red wine, and dark chocolate, play a role in supporting a diverse and healthy gut microbiome.

  - Polyphenols contribute to the overall balance of gut bacteria, fostering a microbiome that is conducive to optimal digestive function.

- **Beta-carotene:**

  - An antioxidant that can be converted into vitamin A, playing a vital role in maintaining the health of the gut lining.

  - Beta-carotene's conversion into vitamin A underscores

its significance in preserving the integrity of the gut lining, essential for overall digestive well-being.

- **Vitamin C (Ascorbic Acid):**

  ○ An antioxidant found in citrus fruits, strawberries, and
  bell peppers, vitamin C supports immune function and
  helps combat oxidative stress in the digestive system.

  ○ Beyond its well-known immune-boosting properties,
  vitamin C contributes to a healthy gut environment by
  neutralizing free radicals.

- **Resveratrol:**

  ○ An antioxidant present in red grapes and berries, resveratrol may have anti-inflammatory effects and, therefore,
  contribute to gut health.

  ○ Resveratrol's inclusion in the diet, often associated with
  moderate red wine consumption, provides an additional
  layer of antioxidant protection for the digestive system.

Incorporating a variety of antioxidant-rich foods into your diet
ensures a comprehensive approach to supporting digestive health, as
these antioxidants collectively contribute to the body's defense against
oxidative challenges.

The Role of Fiber in Gut Health

Fiber is essential for maintaining gut health and overall well-being, impacting digestive processes and the balance of gut microbiota.
There are two types:

- **Insoluble fiber:** Found in whole grains, nuts, seeds, and fruit / vegetable skins, prevents constipation by adding bulk to stool; and

- **Soluble fiber:** Present in oats, legumes, fruits, and vegetables. It undergoes fermentation, producing short-chain fatty acids (SCFAs) with health benefits. SCFAs support the gut barrier, foster beneficial bacteria growth, manage blood sugar levels, and contribute to weight management by inducing satiety.

Certain fiber-rich foods also possess anti-inflammatory properties, potentially reducing gut and body inflammation and lowering the risk of colorectal cancer. To optimize gut health, gradually incorporate a variety of fiber-rich foods, and consider seeking personalized dietary advice from healthcare professionals or registered dietitians (*Dietary Fiber: Essential for a Healthy Diet*, n.d.).

As discussed in previous chapters, prebiotics and probiotics are also crucial for gut health. Probiotics are live beneficial bacteria that enhance gut health by maintaining a balanced microbiota, while prebiotics are non-digestible fibers that nourish these beneficial bacteria, promoting their growth. Together, they contribute to a healthy gut environment.

Even though your gut is an internal organ, and we are still learning a lot about what goes on inside it, the condition of your gut health can significantly impact how you look on the outside. So, the next chapter will focus on the impact of your gut health on your skin as well as your immunity.

Help Transform Lives

REVIEW UNDERSTANDING LEAKY GUT & DIGESTIVE HEALTH!

Unlock the Power of Generosity

"Money can't buy happiness, but sharing knowledge can." - Dr. Ashley Sullivan

People who share knowledge without expecting anything in return tend to lead happier, healthier lives. So, let's aim for that during our time together.

You can make a real difference. To do that, I have a simple question for you ...

Would you be willing to assist someone you haven't met, even if you never received recognition for it? Who is this person, you wonder? They are much like you, or at least like you used to be—seeking information, wanting to make a positive change, and needing guidance.

Our mission is to make the essential information about leaky gut and digestive health accessible to everyone. Everything I do revolves around that mission. And the only way for me to achieve that is by reaching ... well ... everyone.

This is where your help comes in. Most people do, indeed, judge a book by its cover (and its reviews). So, here's my request on behalf of a struggling individual in search of knowledge about digestive health: Please assist that curious learner by leaving a review for this book.

Your gift costs no money and takes less than 60 seconds, but it can change a fellow seeker's life forever. Your review could help ...

- one more person to make informed health decisions.

- one more family adopt healthier habits.

- one more individual regain control of their well-being; or

- one more friend to share valuable insights.

To experience the joy of making a positive impact and genuinely helping someone, all you need to do—in less than 60 seconds—is leave a review.

Simply scan the QR code below to leave your review:

I'm excited to continue guiding you toward understanding leaky gut and digestive health in faster and easier ways than you can imagine. You'll appreciate the practical insights and strategies I'm about to share in the upcoming chapters.

Thank you sincerely. Now, let's return to our journey of discovery. Your biggest supporter, **Dr. Ashley.**

P.S. Fun Fact: If you share valuable information, you become more valuable to others. If you believe this book will help another seeker, pass it along—it might just be the knowledge they're looking for.

CHAPTER SEVEN

The Impact of Gut Health on Skin and Immunity

"*A healthy outside starts from the inside.*" *- Robert Urich*

This chapter focuses on the connection between your gut and skin, explaining how what's happening inside your body can affect how your skin looks and feels. By the end of this chapter, you'll have a better understanding of how keeping your gut healthy can lead to better skin and a stronger immune system.

Understanding the Link between Gut Health and Skin

The relationship between gut health and skin is an intriguing and increasingly acknowledged aspect of overall health. The gut, responsible for digestion and maintaining a balance of bacteria, has a significant impact on various aspects of well-being, including skin condition.

Here are some key points that explain the connection between gut health and skin:

- *Microbiome Influence:* The gut hosts trillions of microorganisms, collectively known as the microbiome, which profoundly affect overall health. A balanced microbiome is linked to healthier skin.

- *Inflammation:* Imbalances in the gut microbiome can lead to inflammation, closely tied to skin conditions like acne and eczema. Chronic gut inflammation may contribute to the development or worsening of skin issues.

- *Nutrient Absorption:* The gut absorbs essential nutrients from food, crucial for skin health. Proper gut function ensures the skin receives the necessary nutrients for repair and maintenance.

- *Immune System Support:* Both the gut and skin are vital components of the immune system. A healthy gut supports a robust immune response, helping the body defend against infections and maintain skin integrity.

- *Holistic Approach:* Holistic skincare approaches recognize the significance of addressing internal factors, like diet and gut health, alongside external factors. Focusing on the gut-skin connection allows for a more comprehensive approach to achieving and maintaining healthy skin.

Maintaining a healthy gut not only aids in digestion but also significantly influences skin health. A balanced and thriving gut microbiome contributes to clearer, healthier skin, while imbalances may result in various skin issues. As our understanding of the gut-skin connection expands, so does the importance of holistic approaches to skincare and overall well-being.

The Gut-Skin Axis and Its Impact on Skin Health

The gut-skin axis represents the intricate connection between the gastrointestinal tract and skin health. This bidirectional communication system involves the gut microbiota, immune system, and various signaling molecules, influencing overall well-being, particularly the condition of the skin.

The gut microbiota, consisting of trillions of microorganisms, plays a crucial role in digestion, nutrient absorption, and immune function. Imbalances in the gut microbiota, referred to as dysbiosis, have been associated with skin conditions such as acne, eczema, and psoriasis.

The gut is a key component of the immune system, and disruptions in the microbiota balance can lead to systemic inflammation, a factor linked to various skin disorders. Nutrient absorption in the gut is essential for maintaining skin health, as nutrients contribute to skin structure, repair, and protection.

The gut-skin axis involves complex interactions, including signaling molecules, stress-related hormones, and inflammatory responses that collectively influence skin well-being. Supporting a healthy gut-skin axis through a balanced diet, hydration, stress management, and avoiding trigger foods can contribute to optimal skin health.

Ongoing research aims to deepen our understanding of these complex connections and their implications for dermatological well-being.

The Role of Inflammation in Gut-Skin Interactions

Inflammation plays a vital role in interactions between the gut and the skin, underscoring the intricate connection between the gastrointestinal tract and skin health. This is because the immune system is a central player in this relationship. Disruptions in the gut can lead to systemic inflammation, which influences various aspects of skin health.

Leaky Gut and Systemic Inflammation:
- Disturbances in gut barrier function, commonly referred to as leaky gut, may arise due to imbalances in the gut microbiota, among other factors. This condition allows the entry of toxins, bacteria, and undigested food particles into the bloodstream.

- The presence of these foreign substances in the bloodstream can trigger an immune response, leading to systemic inflammation. This inflammation may impact the skin, potentially contributing to or exacerbating various skin conditions.

Immune System Activation:
- The gut is a significant part of the immune system, as immune cells in the gut interact with the gut microbiota. Imbalances in the microbiota can activate immune responses, resulting in the release of pro-inflammatory cytokines.

- These cytokines, once in circulation, can influence immune responses throughout the body, potentially affecting the skin and contributing to skin inflammation and conditions, like acne, eczema, or psoriasis.

Skin Conditions Linked to Inflammation:

- Chronic inflammation is a common factor in many skin disorders. Conditions such as acne, rosacea, and psoriasis are characterized by inflammation in the skin.

- In the context of the gut-skin axis, inflammation originating in the gut can contribute to the development or exacerbation of these skin conditions. For example, the release of inflammatory mediators can influence the skin's immune responses and lead to the appearance of skin lesions.

Hormonal Influence:

- The gut-skin axis is interconnected with hormonal regulation. Stress-related hormones, such as cortisol, can be released in response to inflammation or gut disturbances.

- Elevated cortisol levels can contribute to skin issues, potentially increasing sebum production and worsening conditions like acne.

Managing Inflammation for Skin Health:

- Addressing inflammation in the gut is a potential strategy for managing skin conditions. This can involve adopting an anti-inflammatory diet, promoting a healthy gut microbiota through probiotics, and managing stress levels.

- Anti-inflammatory agents and lifestyle changes that promote gut health may contribute to reducing inflammation in the skin and improving overall skin health.

Understanding and addressing the role of inflammation in gut-skin interactions can provide valuable insights for developing strategies to manage and prevent skin conditions, emphasizing the importance of a holistic approach to health that considers both gut and skin well-being (*Gut Bacteria Linked to Inflammatory Skin Disease*, 2021).

Gut-Skin Axis and Its Relationship to Eczema

Eczema, also known as atopic dermatitis, is a chronic inflammatory skin condition characterized by red, itchy, and inflamed skin. While the exact cause of eczema is multifactorial and not fully understood, there is increasing evidence to suggest that the gut-skin axis plays a role in its development and exacerbation.

Several mechanisms contribute to the gut-skin axis and its relationship to eczema:

Immune System Crosstalk: An imbalance in immune responses in the gut can affect the skin and vice versa. Dysregulation in immune function may lead to the development of inflammatory skin conditions like eczema.

Gut Microbiota Influence: The microbial community that makes up the gut microbiota play a crucial role in maintaining immune homeostasis. Changes in the gut microbiota composition, often referred to as dysbiosis, have been associated with inflammatory skin conditions, including eczema.

Intestinal Permeability (Leaky Gut): Increased intestinal permeability can allow the passage of substances from the gut into the bloodstream, triggering immune responses. This phenomenon, commonly referred to as leaky gut, has been linked to skin disorders, including eczema.

Inflammatory Mediators: Inflammatory molecules produced in the gut can circulate throughout the body and influence skin inflammation. Cytokines and other inflammatory mediators may contribute to the development and exacerbation of eczema.

Neuroendocrine Pathways: Communication between the gut and the skin also occurs through neuroendocrine pathways, involving the release of hormones and neurotransmitters. Stress, for example, can impact both the gut and the skin, exacerbating conditions like eczema (Aremu, 2021).

Understanding and addressing the gut-skin axis can help in the management and treatment of eczema. Strategies such as probiotic supplementation, dietary modifications, and lifestyle changes aimed at promoting a healthy gut environment may potentially alleviate eczema symptoms.

However, it's important to note that individual responses to these interventions may vary, and more research is needed to fully elucidate the complex relationship between the gut and skin in the context of eczema.

Psoriasis and Its Connection to Gut Inflammation

Psoriasis is a chronic autoimmune skin disorder characterized by the rapid buildup of skin cells, resulting in thick, red, and scaly patches on the skin. Although the precise cause of psoriasis is not fully understood, emerging evidence suggests a potential link between psoriasis and gut inflammation.

Several factors contribute to the connection between psoriasis and gut inflammation:

Immune System Dysregulation: Psoriasis is considered an immune-mediated disorder. Dysregulation of the immune system can lead to inflammation in various tissues, including the type of inflammation seen in the skin with psoriasis.

Gut Microbiota Imbalance: Studies have suggested that individuals with psoriasis may exhibit alterations in their gut microbiota that are not seen in those without the condition (Polak 2021).

Leaky Gut Syndrome: Some research indicates that individuals with psoriasis may experience higher levels of intestinal permeability (Sikora 2020).

Common Inflammatory Pathways: Psoriasis and inflammatory bowel diseases (IBD), such as Crohn's disease and ulcerative colitis, share some common inflammatory pathways. The inflammatory processes in the gut may influence systemic inflammation, affecting the skin and potentially contributing to the development or exacerbation of psoriasis.

Genetic Factors: Both psoriasis and certain gastrointestinal conditions have genetic components. Shared genetic susceptibility may contribute to the co-occurrence of psoriasis and gut inflammation in some individuals (Paul, 2022).

While the gut-skin axis and the link between psoriasis and gut inflammation are areas of ongoing research, it's important to note that not all individuals with psoriasis experience gastrointestinal issues, and the relationship can vary. Moreover, more research is needed to fully understand the mechanisms underlying this connection and to develop targeted therapeutic strategies.

Individuals with psoriasis may find that lifestyle and dietary changes, such as adopting an anti-inflammatory diet or taking probiotics, can have a positive impact on their skin condition.

However, individuals with psoriasis must consult with healthcare professionals for personalized advice and treatment options tailored to their specific needs.

Understanding the Connection between Gut Health and Aging Skin

Skin aging is a multifaceted process influenced by both intrinsic and extrinsic factors. While factors like sun exposure and genetics have long been recognized as key contributors to aging skin, emerging research suggests that the gut may also play a crucial role in this intricate balance.

Just like in previous discussions about the skin, the connection between gut health and skin aging revolves around the concept of the gut-skin axis. This relationship is mediated by various mechanisms that impact inflammation, nutrient absorption, and microbiota.

As we've seen, gut dysbiosis can trigger systemic inflammation, hastening the breakdown of skin collagen and elastin, ultimately contributing to the formation of wrinkles. Poor gut function may also lead to nutrient deficiencies, expediting the aging process of the skin.

Additionally, imbalances in the gut microbiota influence the immune system, contributing to the development of skin conditions such as acne and eczema, impacting overall skin health and aging.

The gut microbiota plays a role as well in its function of aiding in the regulation of hormones. Stress hormones compromise collagen production and accelerate skin aging.

Promoting gut health through dietary measures, incorporating probiotics, maintaining hydration, managing stress, and avoiding disruptive factors can positively influence skin aging.

Nutrients and Foods for Supporting Skin Elasticity and Preventing Aging

Here's a list of foods that are known to support skin elasticity:

- Fatty Fish: Salmon, mackerel, and other fatty fish are rich in omega-3 fatty acids, which help maintain skin cell membranes and contribute to overall skin health.

- Nuts and Seeds: Almonds, sunflower seeds, and walnuts provide vitamin E, which acts as an antioxidant and helps protect the skin from oxidative stress.

- Citrus Fruits: Oranges, lemons, and grapefruits are high in vitamin C, essential for collagen synthesis and promoting skin elasticity.

- Berries: Blueberries, strawberries, and raspberries are rich in antioxidants that combat free radicals and contribute to anti-aging effects.

- Avocado: This fruit is a good source of healthy fats, including monounsaturated fats, which can help maintain skin moisture and flexibility.

- Leafy Greens: Spinach, kale, and other leafy greens are packed with vitamins (like A, C, and E), minerals, and antioxidants that benefit skin health.

- Tomatoes: Tomatoes contain lycopene, a powerful antioxidant that may protect the skin from sun damage and contribute to skin elasticity.

- Sweet Potatoes: Rich in beta-carotene, sweet potatoes are converted into vitamin A in the body, promoting healthy skin and preventing signs of aging.

- Bell Peppers: Bell peppers, particularly red and yellow ones, are high in vitamin C and antioxidants that support collagen production.

- Broccoli: This vegetable is particularly rich in vitamins C and

K, as well as antioxidants, contributing to overall skin health.

- Green Tea: Green tea contains polyphenols and antioxidants that may help protect the skin from aging and damage caused by free radicals.

- Watermelon: It not only hydrates but also contains lycopene and vitamins A and C, which are beneficial for the skin.

- Eggs: They provide essential amino acids and biotin, contributing to skin health and elasticity.

- Greek Yogurt: Greek yogurt is a good source of protein and probiotics, promoting overall skin health.

- Dark Chocolate: Because it contains flavonoids, it may contribute to skin hydration and protection against UV damage, if enjoyed in moderation.

Remember, maintaining a well-balanced and varied diet, staying hydrated, protecting your skin from excessive sun exposure, and adopting a healthy lifestyle are all crucial factors in supporting skin elasticity and preventing premature aging.

Nutrient-Rich Foods for Skin Health and Gut Nourishment

Consuming nutrient-rich foods is crucial for promoting both skin health and gut nourishment. The relationship between the gut and skin is evident, and a well-balanced diet can positively impact both areas. Below are nutrient-rich foods that contribute to skin health and support a thriving gut. By now, you should recognize a lot of these groups because they are ones that we've talked about in previous chapters. However, it's worth mentioning them again in the context of skin health, as the link between your skin and your gut is so strong.

Probiotic-Rich Foods:
- Yogurt: A natural source of probiotics, yogurt promotes a healthy gut microbiota, aiding digestion and supporting immune function.

- Kefir: This fermented dairy product contains probiotics and can contribute to a diverse and balanced gut microbiota.

Fiber-Rich Foods:
- Whole Grains: Foods like brown rice, quinoa, and oats provide fiber, promoting gut health by supporting the growth of beneficial bacteria.

- Legumes: Beans, lentils, and chickpeas are excellent sources of fiber, helping to maintain gut regularity and support a healthy microbiome.

Fruits and Vegetables:
- Berries: Rich in antioxidants, berries such as blueberries and strawberries help protect the skin from oxidative stress and inflammation.

- Leafy Greens: Spinach, kale, and Swiss chard are high in vitamins, minerals, and fiber, benefiting both gut health and skin radiance.

Fatty Fish:

- Salmon: A source of omega-3 fatty acids, salmon supports skin health by reducing inflammation and promoting skin hydration.

Nuts and Seeds:
- Almonds: Packed with vitamin E, almonds contribute to skin health by protecting against oxidative damage.

- Chia Seeds and Flaxseeds: High in omega-3 fatty acids and fiber, these seeds support gut health and have anti-inflammatory properties beneficial for the skin.

Protein Sources:
- Lean Poultry: Chicken and turkey provide protein necessary for skin repair and collagen synthesis.

- Plant-Based Proteins: Beans, lentils, tofu, and tempeh offer plant-based protein options that support both gut health and skin structure.

Fermented Foods:
- Sauerkraut: Fermented cabbage is rich in probiotics, promoting a healthy gut microbiota.

- Kimchi: A traditional Korean dish, it contains fermented vegetables and beneficial bacteria that contribute to gut health.

Colorful Vegetables:

- Carrots and Sweet Potatoes: Rich in beta-carotene, these vegetables contribute to skin health by supporting collagen production.

- Bell Peppers: High in vitamin C, bell peppers help in collagen synthesis and protect the skin from oxidative stress.

Tea:

- Green tea: Rich in antioxidants, green tea supports skin health by protecting against UV damage and promoting skin elasticity.

Water:

- Staying well-hydrated by drinking plenty of water is crucial for both gut health and skin hydration.

Incorporating a variety of these nutrient-rich foods into your diet supports a symbiotic relationship between gut health and skin vitality. A diverse and balanced diet nourishes the gut microbiota and provides essential nutrients that contribute to healthy, radiant skin.

Antioxidant-Rich Foods and the Benefits of Antioxidants

I'm going to focus on antioxidants in more detail here because they are so essential to the maintenance of skin health and gut nourishment. They do this through counteracting the harmful effects of free radicals in the body and unstable molecules that can cause cellular damage. Free radicals are produced through various processes, including exposure to UV rays, pollution, and normal metabolic activities.

Antioxidant-Rich Foods:

- Berries: Blueberries, strawberries, raspberries, and blackberries are packed with antioxidants like anthocyanins and vitamin C.

- Dark Leafy Greens: Spinach, kale, and Swiss chard contain antioxidants such as lutein, zeaxanthin, and beta-carotene.

- Nuts and Seeds: Almonds, walnuts, chia seeds, and flaxseeds provide vitamin E and other antioxidants.

- Fruits: Citrus fruits, like oranges and grapefruits, contain vitamin C, while avocados provide vitamin E.

- Colorful Vegetables: Carrots, sweet potatoes, and bell peppers are high in beta-carotene and other antioxidants.

- Green Tea: Rich in catechins, green tea has potent antioxidant properties.

- Spices: Turmeric, cinnamon, and ginger contain antioxidants and anti-inflammatory compounds.

- Dark Chocolate: High-quality dark chocolate is rich in flavonoids and can have antioxidant benefits (Jones, n.d.).

Incorporating a variety of antioxidant-rich foods into your diet can be fun. Plus, it brings a balanced and diverse diet for overall well-being. Consulting with a healthcare professional or a nutritionist can provide personalized advice based on individual health needs.

Testimonials

"I struggled with persistent skin issues for years, battling everything

from acne to dullness. Frustrated with conventional skincare remedies, I decided to focus on my gut health. After incorporating probiotic-rich foods and prebiotics into my diet, I noticed a remarkable
change. My skin became clearer and more radiant, and the persistent
redness faded away. The connection between gut health and skin vitality transformed not just my complexion but also my confidence." -
Julia Whiteman (41)

"Eczema has been my constant companion since childhood. Tired
of relying solely on topical treatments, I explored the link between gut
health and skin conditions. By eliminating certain trigger foods and
introducing gut-friendly options like fermented foods, I experienced
a significant reduction in eczema flare-ups. It was a transformative
journey that gave me not just relief from itching but also a newfound
sense of control over my skin health." - **Alex Johnson (19)**

"My adult acne was not just a skin issue but a reflection of hormonal
imbalance. Frustrated with antibiotics and harsh topical treatments, I
decided to address the root cause. Through dietary changes, including
hormone-balancing foods and supplements recommended by a nutritionist, I witnessed a gradual improvement. My skin became less prone
to breakouts, and the painful cystic acne I once battled started to fade
away. It was a reminder that, sometimes, the most effective solutions
come from within." - **Camille Thompson (25)**

"As I approached my forties, signs of aging began affecting my
skin. Intrigued by the gut-skin connection, I revamped my diet with
collagen-rich foods and gut-supporting nutrients. Over time, not only
did my skin regain elasticity, but fine lines also seemed to diminish. I
felt like I had turned back the clock, showcasing that nourishing the
gut could indeed be a natural fountain of youth for the skin." - **Dan
Seth (43)**

Creating a personalized approach to improving gut health for better skin quality involves a combination of dietary, lifestyle, and wellness strategies. Below is a planning tool that you can use to guide the process:

1. Evaluation

Assessment of Gut Health: Evaluate current gut health by examining symptoms and consider professional testing if necessary.

Skin Evaluation: Assess the current state of the skin, noting any issues such as acne or inflammation.

2. Goal Setting

Establish Clear Objectives: Set specific and measurable goals for both gut health and skin improvement.

Timeline Planning: Define a realistic timeline for achieving these goals.

3. Dietary Adjustments

Incorporate Gut-Boosting Foods: Integrate probiotic-rich and prebiotic-rich foods to enhance the gut microbiome.

Hydration Focus: Ensure sufficient water intake to support digestion and skin hydration.

Explore Elimination Diet: Identify and remove potential food triggers through an elimination diet.

4. Supplementation

Probiotic Inclusion: Introduce a quality probiotic supplement to support a healthy gut.

Omega-3 Fatty Acids: Consider adding omega-3 supplements to reduce inflammation and promote skin health.

Collagen Boost: Incorporate collagen supplements to enhance skin elasticity.

5. Lifestyle Modifications

Regular Exercise: Include consistent physical activity to support overall well-being and skin health.

Stress Management Techniques: Implement stress-reducing practices like meditation, yoga, or deep breathing.

Prioritize Adequate Sleep: Ensure 7 to 9 hours of quality sleep to facilitate skin regeneration.

6. Skincare Routine

Gentle Cleansing: Opt for a mild, non-stripping cleanser suitable for your skin type.

Hydration Practices: Use a hydrating moisturizer to maintain skin moisture.

Sun Protection: Apply sunscreen with sufficient SPF to shield the skin from harmful UV rays.

7. Monitoring and Adjustments

Maintain a Journal: Keep a journal to track food intake and symptoms for progress assessment.

Regular Check-Ins: Schedule periodic check-ins to evaluate changes in gut health and skin condition.

Flexibility for Adjustments: Modify the plan based on feedback from your body and progress toward your goals.

8. Professional Guidance

Consult with Experts: Seek advice from a registered dietitian, dermatologist, or healthcare professional for personalized guidance.

Routine Health Check-ups: Schedule regular health check-ups to monitor overall well-being.

Consistency and patience are crucial for success, and adjustments may be necessary as your body responds to the changes. Always consult with healthcare professionals before making significant dietary or lifestyle changes, especially if you have pre-existing health conditions.

CHAPTER EIGHT

Digestive Health through Life's Stages

We will now explore the dynamic connection between digestive health and the various stages of life. From early childhood to the golden years of aging, our digestive systems undergo significant transformations that profoundly impact our overall well-being.

Did you know that, according to research, from infancy, the choices made regarding early feeding practices can significantly impact gut health? The composition of the gut microbiome is particularly influenced by factors such as the types of foods introduced early on and the methods of feeding.

These early influences play a crucial role in shaping a healthy and diverse gut microbiota in infants, with potential long-term effects on digestive health and overall well-being throughout various life stages. Recognizing the importance of these early choices is essential for fostering a resilient and balanced gut microbiome right from the earliest stages of life.

Nurturing a Healthy Gut from Birth

Promoting gut health in childhood is crucial for overall well-being, as the early years establish the foundation for a resilient digestive system. Nurturing a healthy gut from birth is particularly important, as it can have lasting effects on a child's health and development. As we explore the wonders of gut health, know that every feeding choice contributes to your child's well-being and embrace the unique journey you've chosen for your little one. Here are key considerations in understanding and supporting gut health in childhood:

Microbial Colonization at Birth:

The process of microbial colonization begins at birth, where a newborn's gut is populated by microorganisms from the mother, the environment, and the delivery method. Vaginal births expose infants to the mother's microbiota, while cesarean births may result in a different microbial composition. Take comfort in knowing that both paths, although different, play a crucial role in establishing a diverse and resilient gut microbiome.

The Role of Breastfeeding:

Breastfeeding also contributes significantly to the establishment of a diverse and beneficial gut microbiome. Breast milk is rich in nutrients and bioactive compounds that support the growth of beneficial bacteria in the infant's gut. It contains prebiotics, probiotics, and antibodies that contribute to the development of a robust immune system and a healthy gut microbiome. Breastfeeding is recognized for its role in reducing the risk of various digestive issues and promoting optimal gut health in early childhood. While breastfeeding has its unique benefits, formula feeding comes with its own set of nurturing moments. Although breast milk is a powerhouse of nutrients and bioactive compounds, formula feeding also provides a reliable source of nutrition tailored to your baby's needs.

Introduction of Solid Foods:

As a child transitions to solid foods, a diverse diet becomes crucial for nurturing a healthy gut. Introducing a variety of fruits, vegetables, whole grains, and other nutrient-rich foods supports the growth of a diverse microbial community. Avoiding excessive use of antibiotics and processed foods is also essential, as these factors can disrupt the balance of gut bacteria.

Importance of Fiber:

Dietary fiber plays a key role in promoting gut health by acting as a prebiotic, providing fuel for beneficial bacteria. Including fiber-rich foods in a child's diet, such as fruits, vegetables, and whole grains, helps maintain a healthy balance of gut microbiota, aiding in digestion and nutrient absorption.

Proactive Health Measures:

Ensuring good hygiene practices, promoting physical activity, and encouraging healthy sleeping patterns are proactive measures that contribute to maintaining a healthy gut in childhood. These practices help preserve the delicate balance of the gut microbiome and support the development of a robust immune system.

Birth Methods and Gut Considerations

An impacted gut can lead to colic and congestion.

An impacted gut in babies can lead to colic and congestion, due to factors like constipation, gut microbiome imbalance, feeding issues, and reflux. Constipation causes abdominal discomfort and contributes to colic, while an imbalanced gut microbiome can result in gas and digestive discomfort. Introducing new formulas or sudden dietary changes may also impact the gut. Gastroesophageal reflux (GERD) associated with an impacted gut can cause congestion and respiratory issues. Probiotics, dietary adjustments, and maintaining hydration are strategies to address and prevent these issues.

C-section babies will need early prebiotic and probiotic support.

C-section babies, those delivered through cesarean section, can benefit from early pre and probiotic support to encourage optimal gut health. Unlike infants born through natural delivery, C-section babies do not have the opportunity to be exposed to their mother's vaginal and fecal microbes, which are essential for seeding their gut with beneficial bacteria.

- *Absence of Vaginal Microbial Transfer:* C-section births lack exposure to the beneficial microbes found in the birth canal, potentially affecting the initial composition of the infant's gut microbiota.

- *Significance of Early Microbial Colonization:* Early microbial colonization is crucial for developing a diverse and balanced gut microbiome, influencing various aspects of health such as immune function, metabolism, and digestion.

- *Probiotics for C-section Babies:* Administering probiotics, live beneficial bacteria, may help establish a healthy gut microbiome in C-section babies. Commonly used probiotic strains for infants include Lactobacillus and Bifidobacterium.

- *Prebiotics to Support Probiotics:* The introduction of prebiotics—non-digestible fibers promoting the growth of beneficial bacteria—can support the effectiveness of probiotics.

- *Potential Health Benefits:* Early pre and probiotic supplementation in C-section babies could potentially reduce the risk of conditions such as allergies, asthma, and other immune-related disorders. Improved gut health may contribute to better nutrient absorption and overall well-being.

- *Breastfeeding as a Natural Source:* Breast milk itself contains beneficial microbes and serves as a natural source of prebiotics, supporting the establishment of a healthy gut microbiome in infants.

- *Formula feeding as an Alternative:* Formula brings its own set of nurturing moments, offering a dependable source of nutrition that is customized to meet your baby's requirements.

All in all, while additional research is necessary, early pre and probiotic support for C-section babies may help compensate for the lack of natural microbial exposure during birth.

Parent Testimonials

"I observed a fascinating connection between my child's mood and digestive health. When we incorporated probiotic-rich foods into their diet, they seemed happier and more content. It was a personal realization of the potential link between early gut health and the development of a positive mood in infants." - **Emily & Patrick**

"Dealing with an infant suffering from reflux was challenging. After consulting with a healthcare professional, we introduced probiotics into our baby's routine, leading to a noticeable reduction in reflux symptoms." - **Jane & Isaac**

"Having children born through both C-section and natural births, we noticed distinct differences in their gut health. Our child born through natural birth appeared to have a more robust digestive system and experienced fewer tummy troubles." - **Ilena & Jack**

"We faced the challenging period of dealing with a colicky baby. It was tough to see our little one in distress. After consulting with our healthcare professional, we decided to try probiotics. Gradually, we noticed a reduction in colic symptoms, and our baby seemed more at ease." - **Kate & Mark**

Further Strategies to Support Gut Health in Newborns and Babies

- *Fiber for Moms*: Maintain a diet rich in fiber during pregnancy by incorporating fruits, grains, nuts, legumes, and vegetables.

- *Delayed First Bath*: Postponing the first bath provides multiple benefits, including enhanced bonding and protection against infections.

Probiotics for Moms: Mothers can consider prenatal probiotics for potential benefits.

A Young Girl's Journey through Intestinal Challenges

Mia's story unfolded in a small town, where she faced the unique challenge of gastroschisis. Born with her intestines outside her tiny body, Mia found solace at Lucile Packard Children's Hospital at Stanford. Lily, her adoptive mother, became a pillar of strength in navigating the complexities of intestinal failure and total parenteral nutrition (TPN) dependence during Mia's early years.

The gradual transformation in Mia's life was marked by the delicate dance of medical care and Lily's unwavering dedication. Specialists at the hospital guided caring for Mia, ensuring her nutritional needs were met through personalized plans.

Mia's journey toward independence from TPN was a remarkable testament to adaptation. She now joyfully partakes in family meals from minimal food intake as a toddler. Regular checkups, orchestrated by a dedicated healthcare team, fine-tune Mia's nutrition plan, ensuring her growth and well-being.

Lily's goal mirrored the determination of many caregivers—to guide Mia toward independence from TPN. The support Mia found in her journey through personalized eating plans, enhanced by a tenacious spirit, ensured her success. Today, Mia, a spirited eight-year-old, thrives with reduced TPN support, embodying resilience and triumph (Nichols, 2020).

Exploring Dietary Habits for Optimal Gut Health in Kids

Here are some tips on how you can improve gut health in your children:

- Emphasize breastfeeding during the initial six months and continue as long as possible to establish a healthy gut flora.

- Maintain a balanced diet with a variety of soluble and insoluble fiber-rich foods like quinoa, oats, lentils, and beans.

- Limit the intake of fatty foods, junk food, caffeinated beverages, and candy. Instead, focus on incorporating healthy fats and high-fiber foods for optimal digestion.

- Include easily digestible lean meats, such as chicken, to support improved digestion and nutrient absorption.

- Integrate probiotics into their diet through natural sources, like yogurt, kefir, and sauerkraut, or consider a pediatrician-recommended probiotic supplement.

- Choose small, frequent meals to facilitate easier consumption, provide sustained energy, and maintain continuous digestive system activity.

- Ensure proper hydration with water or alternatives like fruit-infused water, fresh fruit juices, tender coconut water, melons, and cucumbers.

- Encourage regular physical activity, including exercises and specific yoga poses, to promote overall well-being and stimulate the digestive system.

- Use antibiotics judiciously, avoiding unnecessary courses to preserve long-term gut health.

- Promote outdoor exposure to germs for enhanced gut and immune health, emphasizing basic hygiene without over-sanitizing to build natural immunity (*10 Tips to Maintain a Healthy Gut in Kids*, n.d.).

Common Digestive Challenges in Children and How to Address Them

Children may encounter a range of digestive challenges, including issues like constipation, diarrhea, GERD, food allergies, IBS, lactose intolerance, celiac disease, bloating, gas, and overeating.

Managing these concerns often involves dietary adjustments, such as ensuring sufficient fiber intake and avoiding trigger foods. Lifestyle factors, including hydration, regular physical activity, and consistent routines, are crucial for digestive health.

Additionally, seeking guidance from healthcare professionals is vital for accurate diagnosis and personalized management plans tailored to the child's needs. Encouraging mindful eating habits and providing a balanced diet contribute to overall digestive well-being, supporting a healthy foundation for children's growth and development.

Women, Hormones, and Gut Changes: Why Your Gut Gets Worse during Your Cycle

Women undergo natural hormonal fluctuations during their menstrual cycle, mainly involving estrogen and progesterone. These changes can influence digestive function. In the first half of the cycle, estrogen levels rise, peaking before ovulation, while the second half sees increased progesterone to prepare for potential pregnancy. These hormonal shifts can affect the gut in various ways:

- *Slowed Digestion:* Elevated progesterone relaxes smooth muscle tissue, including the digestive tract muscles, leading to slower transit times and feelings of bloating or constipation.

- *Water Retention:* Hormonal changes may disturb water balance, causing some women to experience bloating and discomfort due to water retention.

- *Sensitivity to Pain:* Hormones influence pain perception, potentially making some women more sensitive to abdominal discomfort or cramping during their menstrual period.

- *Microbiome Changes:* Hormonal fluctuations can impact the gut microbiome, affecting the composition and activity of microorganisms in the digestive tract. This can potentially lead to gut symptoms that include digestive discomfort, irregular bowel movements, increased food sensitivity, anxiety, stress, or mood swings.

- *Increased Sensitivity:* Some women may experience heightened gut sensitivity during their menstrual cycle, resulting in increased discomfort or symptoms associated with conditions like irritable bowel syndrome (IBS) (*Gut Health and Your Menstrual Cycle: What Women Need to Know*, 2022).

Individual responses to these changes vary. While some women may not notice significant digestive alterations, others may experience pronounced symptoms.

Managing these effects involves maintaining a healthy diet, staying hydrated, engaging in regular physical activity, and considering stress reduction techniques. Dietary adjustments and lifestyle modifications can often alleviate symptoms associated with hormonal fluctuations, promoting better digestive health.

Seniors Experiencing Improved Quality of Life Through Gut Health Support

"Seeking a solution to my digestive issues, I consulted with a nutritionist who recommended focusing on gut health. I adjusted my diet, incorporating more fiber-rich foods and probiotics. As time passed, I noticed a remarkable improvement in my digestion, with reduced discomfort and increased energy levels. Now, I happily share my personal success story, emphasizing the transformative impact of prioritizing gut health on my overall well-being." - **Elsa (75)**

"I embraced a holistic approach to gut health with guidance from my healthcare provider. By introducing fermented foods and prebiotics into my diet, I experienced gradual but significant positive changes. My digestive issues subsided, and I discovered a renewed sense of well-being. Now, I encourage others in my age group to prioritize gut health, believing it's never too late to embark on a journey toward improved vitality." - **James (68)**

Understanding Changes in the Gut as We Age

As we age, several changes occur in the gut. Muscle strength and coordination decline, leading to slower digestion and potential constipation. Digestive enzyme production also decreases, which in turn affects nutrient absorption. In addition to this, the gut microbiome undergoes alterations, and the intestinal lining may thin, making the gut more susceptible to irritation. Plus, stomach acid production decreases, impacting nutrient absorption. The risk of gastrointestinal disorders, like diverticulosis and IBS, also increases with age.

To support gut health, maintain a balanced diet that includes plenty of fiber, stay hydrated, exercise regularly, consider probiotics, and undergo regular health check-ups for early detection and management of digestive conditions.

Nutrition for Healthy Aging

"At seventy-two, I faced digestive discomfort affecting my daily life. After consulting a nutritionist, I embraced a gut-friendly diet rich in fiber, fruits, and probiotics. The change was remarkable. Gradually, my digestive issues eased, and I regained vitality. Now, at seventy-five, I enjoy each day with newfound comfort, all thanks to prioritizing my gut health through simple dietary changes." - **Clara**

"In my late sixties, digestive challenges made me apprehensive about enjoying my golden years. With guidance from a healthcare professional, I adopted a balanced diet with whole grains and fermented foods. The impact on my gut health was significant—less bloating, improved regularity, and increased energy. Now, at seventy-two, I savor life's moments with a renewed sense of well-being, grateful for the positive changes a gut-friendly diet brought to my daily life." - **Vivien**

Dietary Recommendations for Maintaining Gut Health in the Elderly

Maintaining gut health is crucial for individuals aged fifty and above due to changes in the digestive system with age. Here are specific dietary recommendations tailored for older adults:

- *Fiber-Rich Foods:* Prioritize a diet high in fiber from sources like whole grains, fruits, vegetables, and legumes to prevent constipation and support digestive health.

- *Probiotics and Fermented Foods:* Include probiotic-rich foods, such as yogurt, kefir, sauerkraut, and kimchi, to introduce beneficial bacteria to the gut, aiding in digestion and helping to maintain a balanced microbiome.

- *Adequate Hydration:* Ensure sufficient water intake throughout the day to support the mucous layer in the intestines, preventing constipation and promoting overall digestive well-being.

- *Prebiotic-Rich Foods:* Incorporate prebiotic foods, like garlic, onions, bananas, and asparagus, into meals to act as fuel for beneficial gut bacteria, promoting their growth and activity.

- *Lean Proteins:* Choose lean protein sources, such as poultry, fish, and plant-based proteins, which are easier on the digestive system and contribute to overall gut health.

- *Whole Grains:* Choose whole grains like brown rice, quinoa, and whole wheat for their fiber and nutrient content, supporting digestive health and regularity.

- *Limit Processed Foods:* Reduce the consumption of processed foods, focusing on whole, minimally processed options to avoid additives that can disrupt the balance of the gut microbiome.

- *Moderate Fat Intake:* Maintain a balanced intake of healthy fats from sources like olive oil, avocados, and nuts to support nutrient absorption and contribute to overall gut function.

- *Diverse Diet:* Aim for a diverse and well-balanced diet, including a variety of fruits, vegetables, whole grains, and proteins to promote a diverse microbiome crucial for gut health.

- *Consult with a Healthcare Professional:* Given that individual dietary needs can vary, older adults should consult healthcare professionals or registered dietitians for personalized recommendations, considering specific health conditions, medications, and dietary preferences.

- *Monitor Lactose Intake:* Be mindful of lactose intolerance that may develop with age, monitor dairy intake, and consider lactose-free alternatives if necessary (*Nutrition Needs When You're Over 65*, n.d.).

By incorporating these age-specific dietary recommendations, individuals aged fifty and above can actively promote their gut health, enhance digestive function, and contribute to overall well-being. It's advisable to approach dietary changes gradually and seek professional guidance for personalized advice tailored to individual health needs.

This chapter focused on how our gut, like any other organ, can behave differently at every stage of our life. From childhood to our older years, the way our gut behaves can change. Next up is the epilogue, where you can find encouragement from some amazing success stories.

Real Stories of Gut Transformation

"I battled persistent bloating and irregular bowel habits that significantly impacted my daily life. Consulting with a healthcare professional, I discovered an imbalanced gut microbiome. Taking charge of my gut health, I adopted a diet rich in fiber, probiotics, and prebiotics. Gradually, my symptoms were alleviated, and I restored balance to my digestion. Today, I maintain my gut health with a diverse and wholesome diet." - **Olivia (55)**

"I faced ongoing indigestion and discomfort following meals. A thorough examination revealed reduced stomach acid production as the root cause. Making dietary adjustments, I opted for smaller, more frequent meals and introduced digestive enzymes. This approach proved successful as my symptoms improved, allowing me to savor meals without prior discomfort." - **James (60)**

"I confronted challenges with constipation and sluggish digestion. Identifying a deficiency in dietary fiber, I revamped my eating habits, embracing whole grains, fruits, and vegetables. This dietary shift notably enhanced my bowel regularity, underscoring the significance of a fiber-rich diet for gut health."- **Sophie (27)**

"I experienced recurring digestive upset and bloating, attributing it to an imbalance in my gut microbiome. Taking proactive steps, I incorporated probiotic-rich foods and supplements into my daily routine. Over time, my gut balance was restored, and I found relief from digestive discomfort." - **Nathan (32)**

"I dealt with intermittent constipation and low energy levels. Identifying inadequate hydration as a contributing factor, I prioritized water intake, especially during meals. This simple adjustment resulted in improved digestion, heightened energy, and an overall sense of well-being. My commitment to hydration became a cornerstone for maintaining my gut health." - **Anna (41)**

Conclusion

We are now wrapping up our exploration of digestive health. We've delved into various aspects, from understanding digestion and unraveling digestive disorders to exploring the gut-brain connection and making informed lifestyle choices for digestive wellness. Our journey has covered healing herbs, the impact of gut health on skin and immunity, and considerations for digestive well-being through different life stages. The epilogue serves as a testament to the practical application of the insights provided throughout this book.

The central message resounds clearly: the well-being of our gut profoundly influences our overall health. The crux of our journey is the importance of nurturing and maintaining a healthy gut for a thriving life. It goes beyond mere dietary choices; it encompasses the profound impact that such choices have on our physical, mental, and emotional health.

The three real-life stories shared in the introduction illustrated the widespread challenges faced by individuals neglecting their gut health. Sandra, Jenny, and Claire encountered various health issues, underscoring the far-reaching consequences of an unhealthy gut.

Returning to these stories, we witnessed the transformative power of knowledge and intentional choices. Sandra found balance in her hectic life by prioritizing nourishing foods and managing stress. Jenny regained vitality, overcoming stomach issues and restoring her well-being through mindful dietary changes. Claire, a professional with a demanding lifestyle, took control of her health through balanced meals and physical activity.

These success stories highlight a fundamental truth: every small choice impacts our gut and, consequently, our future health and well-being. Change, no matter how small, can lead to significant transformations. The journey toward a healthier gut begins with the smallest, easiest steps. The very first? A commitment to making mindful choices today.

As you embark on your journey to digestive wellness, remember the lessons learned within these pages. Embrace the power of informed decisions, mindful nourishment, and the remarkable connection between your gut and overall health. Your gut is not just a digestive organ; it's a cornerstone of your well-being.

Consider this a call to action: Start today, armed with newfound knowledge and inspired by the success stories within! Your gut transformation awaits, and your future self will undoubtedly thank you for this investment in your health. If this journey has resonated with you, share your thoughts and experiences. Your genuine reflections may inspire others to take the first step toward a healthier digestive system. Here's to your journey into a vibrant, gut-healthy life!

Share the Knowledge

Now that you have all the tools to embark on your gut-healing journey, it's time to pay it forward and guide other readers to the same transformative knowledge.

By sharing your honest thoughts about this book on Amazon, you're not just leaving a review; you're illuminating the path for fellow readers. Your review becomes a compass, directing others to the information they seek and fostering their passion for understanding leaky gut and digestive health.

Your contribution is priceless. The passion for self-education and understanding thrives when we share our newfound knowledge—and you're playing a pivotal role in making that happen.

Click here to leave your review on Amazon.

Thank you for being an integral part of this mission. The journey of self-education and understanding continues when we generously share our insights with others.

With gratitude,

Dr. Ashley Sullivan, PharmD, RPh, MBA

Ways to Connect:

Follow Dr. Ashley Sullivan, PharmD on Facebook, link below

https://www.facebook.com/profile.php?id=100092716005488

Website https://ashleysullivanonline.com/

Join her FREE Facebook group "Compassionate Care and Holistic Advocacy with Dr. Ashley", link below.

https://www.facebook.com/groups/907620087038942

Gut Friendly Recipes

Quinoa Parfait

Ingredients:

- ½ cup cooked quinoa

- ½ cup Greek yogurt

- 1 tablespoon honey

- ¼ cup fresh berries (blueberries, strawberries, or raspberries)

- 1 tablespoon chia seeds

- 1 tablespoon chopped nuts (almonds, walnuts, or pistachios)

Instructions:

- In a bowl, layer half of the cooked quinoa.

- Add a layer of Greek yogurt on top of the quinoa.

- Drizzle honey over the yogurt layer.

- Sprinkle fresh berries evenly over the honey layer.

- Add the remaining quinoa on top of the berries.

- Sprinkle chia seeds and chopped nuts over the final quinoa layer.

- Serve chilled and enjoy this nutritious and gut-supportive breakfast parfait.

Grilled Salmon with Quinoa and Roasted Vegetables

Ingredients:

- 1 salmon fillet

- 1 cup cooked quinoa

- 1 cup mixed vegetables (bell peppers, zucchini, cherry tomatoes)

- 1 tablespoon olive oil

- 1 teaspoon lemon juice

- Salt and pepper to taste

- Fresh herbs for garnish (parsley or dill)

Instructions:

- Preheat the grill or oven to medium-high heat.

- Season the salmon fillet with salt, pepper, and lemon juice.

- In a bowl, toss the mixed vegetables with olive oil, salt, and pepper.

- Grill or roast the salmon fillet and mixed vegetables until cooked through.

- Place a serving of cooked quinoa on a plate.

- Top with grilled salmon and roasted vegetables.

- Garnish with fresh herbs.

- Serve warm and savor this satisfying and digestion-friendly main course.

Ginger Turmeric Tea

Ingredients:

- 1-inch piece of fresh ginger, sliced

- 1 teaspoon ground turmeric

- 1 tablespoon honey

- 1 lemon wedge

- 2 cups hot water

Instructions:

- In a teapot, combine ginger slices, ground turmeric, and honey.

- Squeeze the lemon wedge into the mixture.

- Pour hot water over the ingredients.

- Let it steep for 5-7 minutes.

- Strain the tea into a cup.

- Enjoy this soothing and gut-supportive beverage for a refreshing snack.

Probiotic-Rich Smoothie

Ingredients:

- 1 cup Greek yogurt

- 1 ripe banana

- 1/2 cup mixed berries (blueberries, strawberries, or raspberries)

- 1 tablespoon honey

- 1/2 cup kefir

Directions:

- Place all ingredients in a blender.

- Blend until smooth.

- Pour into a glass and enjoy your probiotic-rich smoothie!

Quinoa Salad with Fermented Veggies

Ingredients:

- 1 cup cooked quinoa

- 1/2 cup fermented vegetables (kimchi, sauerkraut)

- 1 cucumber, diced

- Lemon-tahini dressing (1 tablespoon tahini, juice of 1 lemon, salt)

Directions:

- In a bowl, combine quinoa, fermented veggies, and diced cucumber.

- In a small bowl, whisk together the lemon-tahini dressing.

- Pour the dressing over the quinoa mixture and toss to combine.

Ginger Turmeric Carrot Soup

Ingredients:

- 4 cups carrots, chopped

- 1 tablespoon fresh ginger, grated

- 1 tablespoon fresh turmeric, grated

- 4 cups vegetable broth

- 1 cup coconut milk

- Salt and black pepper to taste

Directions:

- In a pot, combine carrots, ginger, turmeric, and vegetable broth.

- Bring to a boil, then simmer until carrots are tender.

- Blend the mixture until smooth, then return to the pot.

- Stir in coconut milk and season with salt and pepper.

Salmon and Avocado Salad:
Ingredients:
- 2 cups mixed greens

- 6 oz grilled salmon, flaked

- 1 avocado, sliced

- Cherry tomatoes, halved

- Olive oil and lemon dressing

Directions:
- Arrange mixed greens on a plate.

- Top with grilled salmon, avocado slices, and cherry tomatoes.

- Drizzle with olive oil and lemon dressing.

Chickpea and Vegetable Stir-Fry
Ingredients:
- 1 can chickpeas, drained and rinsed

- Mixed vegetables (bell peppers, broccoli, snap peas)

- 2 cloves garlic, minced

- 2 tablespoons tamari or soy sauce

- 1 tablespoon sesame oil

Directions:

- In a pan, sauté garlic in sesame oil.

- Add mixed vegetables and chickpeas, stir-fry until tender.

- Pour tamari or soy sauce, toss until well-coated.

Blueberry Chia Pudding

Ingredients:

- 1/4 cup chia seeds

- 1 cup almond milk

- 1/2 cup blueberries (fresh or frozen)

- 1 tablespoon honey

- Almonds for topping

Directions:

- In a jar, mix chia seeds and almond milk. Refrigerate for a few hours or overnight.

- Layer with blueberries and drizzle honey.

- Top with almonds before serving.

Roasted Turmeric Cauliflower

Ingredients:

- 1 head cauliflower, cut into florets

- 2 tablespoons olive oil

- 1 teaspoon turmeric

- 1/2 teaspoon cumin

- Salt and pepper to taste

Directions:
- Toss cauliflower in olive oil, turmeric, cumin, salt, and pepper.

- Roast in the oven until golden brown.

Gut-Healing Green Smoothie
Ingredients:
- 1 cup kale or spinach

- 1/2 cucumber

- 1/2 banana

- 1/2 cup pineapple chunks

- 1 cup coconut water

Directions:
- Blend all ingredients until smooth.

- Pour into a glass and enjoy your green smoothie.

Feel free to adjust the quantities and ingredients based on your preferences and dietary needs. These recipes aim to provide nourishment and support for a healthy gut!

Medications for Digestive Disorders

Embarking on a journey toward optimal gut health involves a comprehensive approach, with lifestyle playing a pivotal role. My primary focus is to uncover and address the root causes of digestive issues, promoting holistic well-being. However, I recognize that symptoms can sometimes disrupt your daily life and well-being, necessitating additional support. As a pharmacist, this book wouldn't be complete without discussing all the options.

In this section, I provide valuable insights into medications commonly used to address digestive concerns. It's essential to approach medication as a complementary tool alongside lifestyle changes, aiming for a balanced and personalized approach to enhance your digestive wellness. Let's explore the medications frequently employed in the realm of digestive health, understanding their roles and how they can contribute to your journey toward a healthier gut.

Antacids:

- Examples include calcium carbonate (found in Tums) and a combination of aluminum hydroxide/magnesium hydroxide (Maalox). Other options are Pepto-Bismol, Rolaids, and Mylanta.

- These medications alleviate symptoms of heartburn and indigestion by neutralizing excess stomach acid.

Proton Pump Inhibitors (PPIs):
- Examples of PPIs are Omeprazole (sold as Prilosec), Esomeprazole (Nexium), and Lansoprazole (Prevacid). Other brands include Protonix, Aciphex, and Dexilant.

- PPIs are used for the short-term treatment of gastroesophageal reflux disease (GERD) and peptic ulcers, as they reduce the production of stomach acid.

H2 Blockers (Histamine-2 Receptor Antagonists):
- Examples of H2 blockers are Ranitidine (Zantac), Famotidine (Pepcid), and Cimetidine (Tagamet).

- These medications relieve symptoms of heartburn and indigestion by blocking histamine, which in turn reduces the production of stomach acid.

Antispasmodics:
- Examples of antispasmodics include Dicyclomine (Bentyl) and Hyoscyamine (Levsin).

- These medications help alleviate abdominal cramps and spasms by relaxing the smooth muscles in the digestive tract.

Laxatives:

- Examples of laxatives include Psyllium (Metamucil), Bisacodyl (Dulcolax), Polyethylene Glycol (Miralax), and Senokot.

- These medications relieve constipation by promoting bowel movements.

Antidiarrheals:

- Examples include Loperamide (Imodium) and Bismuth Subsalicylate (found in Pepto-Bismol).

- They are used to slow down bowel movements and reduce inflammation, providing relief from diarrhea.

Antiemetics (for nausea and vomiting):

- Examples are Ondansetron (Zofran), Metoclopramide (Reglan), and Dimenhydrinate (Dramamine).

- These medications suppress nausea and vomiting.

Stool Softeners:

- Docusate (Colace) is often used.

- This medication relieves difficulty passing stools by adding moisture to them, making them easier to pass.

Prokinetic Agents (to improve gastrointestinal motility):

- Examples include Metoclopramide (Reglan) and Domperidone.

- These medications enhance gastrointestinal motility.

Digestive Enzymes:

- Examples include Pancrelipase (Creon, Pancreaze) and Lactase supplements (Lactaid).

- These medications aid in the digestion of nutrients and are used for digestive enzyme deficiencies.

Antiflatulents:
- Examples include Simethicone (Gas-X) and Charcoal (activated charcoal).

- These medications break down gas bubbles, providing relief from gas and bloating.

Gastrointestinal Protective Agents:
- An example is Sucralfate (Carafate).

- This medication forms a protective barrier on the stomach lining, providing relief from peptic ulcers and gastritis.

Hepatoprotective Agents (for liver health):
- Examples include Ursodiol (Actigall) and Silymarin (Milk Thistle).

- These medications support and protect liver function.

Antiulcer Agents (for preventing and treating ulcers):
- Examples include Misoprostol (Cytotec) and Rebamipide (Mucosta).

- These medications promote healing and reduce the formation of peptic ulcers.

Gallstone Dissolving Agents:
- An example is Ursodiol (Actigall).

- This medication is used to dissolve cholesterol-based gall-stones.

Bile Acid Sequestrants (for cholesterol management):

- Examples include Cholestyramine (Questran) and Cole-sevelam (Welchol).

- These medications reduce cholesterol absorption by binding to bile acids.

Anti-inflammatory Agents (for inflammatory bowel diseases):

- Examples include Mesalamine (Asacol, Pentasa) and Pred-nisone.

- These medications reduce inflammation in the digestive tract, providing relief from inflammatory bowel diseases.

Antibiotics (for bacterial infections in the GI tract):

- Examples include Ciprofloxacin (Cipro) and Metronidazole (Flagyl).

- These medications are used to treat bacterial infections in the gastrointestinal tract.

Immunosuppressants (for autoimmune conditions of the digestive system):

- Examples include Azathioprine (Imuran) and Infliximab (Remicade).

- These medications suppress the immune response and are used to treat autoimmune conditions affecting the digestive system.

Opioid Receptor Antagonists (for opioid-induced constipation):

- Examples include Naloxegol (Movantik) and Methylnal-trexone (Relistor).

- These medications block the constipating effects of opioids and provide relief from constipation caused by opioid use.

Suspected Gut-Unfriendly Medications

The following list of medications are often suspected to have potential effects on gut health based on common knowledge. Please note that individual reactions may vary, and it's important to consult with a healthcare professional for personalized advice. Here are some medications that are often discussed in relation to potential impacts on gut health:

- Antibiotics: They can disrupt the balance of gut bacteria by killing both harmful and beneficial microbes.

- Non-Steroidal Anti-Inflammatory Drugs (NSAIDs): Regular use of NSAIDs, such as ibuprofen and aspirin, may lead to irritation and damage to the gastrointestinal tract.

- Proton Pump Inhibitors (PPIs): These drugs reduce stomach acid production and may affect the balance of gut bacteria.

- Steroids: Long-term use of corticosteroids can impact the gut microbiota.

- Birth Control Pills: Hormonal contraceptives may influence gut health in some individuals.

- Antidepressants: Some antidepressants may have effects on

the gut microbiota.

- Immunosuppressants: Medications that suppress the immune system may have an impact on gut health.

It's important to emphasize that the impact of medications on gut health can vary from person to person, and in many cases, the benefits of these medications may outweigh any potential negative effects on gut health. If you have concerns about the medications, you are taking and their impact on your gut health, it's best to discuss them with your healthcare provider. They can provide personalized advice based on your specific health needs and conditions.

References

1. Anguita-Ruiz A, Aguilera CM, Gil Á. Genetics of Lactose Intolerance: An Updated Review and Online Interactive World Maps of Phenotype and Genotype Frequencies. Nutrients. 2020 Sep 3;12(9):2689. doi: 10.3390/nu12092689. PMID: 32899182; PMCID: PMC7551416.

2. Appleton J. (2018). The Gut-Brain Axis: Influence of Microbiota on Mood and Mental Health. Integrative medicine (Encinitas, Calif.), 17(4), 28–32.

3. Appleton J. (2018). The Gut-Brain Axis: Influence of Microbiota on Mood and Mental Health. *Integrative medicine (Encinitas, Calif.)*, *17*(4), 28–32.

4. Barbara Bolen, P. (2022, September 6). *Why enzymes are an important part of your digestive system*. Verywell Health. https://www.verywellhealth.com/what-are-digestive-enzymes-1945036

5. Barbara Bolen, P. (2022a, September 6). *Why enzymes are an important part of your digestive system*. Verywell Health. https://www.verywellhealth.com/what-are-digesti ve-enzymes-1945036

6. Case-Lo, C. (2020, November 5). *How does serotonin in the brain affect your bowels?*. Healthline. https://www.healthli ne.com/health/irritable-bowel-syndrome/serotonin-effects

7. *Constipation   symptoms   and   treat- ments*.   NHS   inform.   (1BC,   November 30). https://www.nhsinform.scot/illnesses-and-condition s/stomach-liver-and-gastrointestinal-tract/constipation

8. Courtney E. Ackerman, MA. (2023, September 22). *Mindfulness-Based Stress Reduction: The Ultimate MBSR Guide*. PositivePsychology.com. https://positivepsychology.com/ mindfulness-based-stress-reduction-mbsr/

9. Department of Health & Human Services. (1999, May 18). *Crohn's disease and ulcerative colitis*. Better Health Channel. https://www.betterhealth.vic.gov.au/health/con ditionsandtreatments/crohns-disease-and-ulcerative-colitis

10. Edermaniger, L. (2022, March 9). *How to improve gut health: 16 simple hacks for your gut in 2022*. Atlas Biomed blog | Take control of your health with no-nonsense news on lifestyle, gut microbes and ge- netics. https://atlasbiomed.com/blog/16-easy-hacks-to-en hance-your-gut-health-every-day-in-2020/

11. Evenepoel, P., Dejongh, S., Verbeke, K., & Meijers, B. (2020).

The Role of Gut Dysbiosis in the Bone–Vascular Axis in Chronic Kidney Disease. Toxins, 12(5), 285. https://doi.o rg/10.3390/toxins12050285

12. *Foods linked to better brainpower*. Harvard Health. (2021, March 6). https://www.health.harvard.edu/healthbeat/fo ods-linked-to-better-brainpower

13. *Gastroesophageal   reflux   disease   (GERD)*. Johns   Hopkins   Medicine.   (n.d.) . https://www.hopkinsmedicine.org/health/conditions-an d-diseases/gastroesophageal-reflux-disease-gerd

14. Gina Simmons Schneider, Ph. D. (2022, August 26). *This is exactly how anxiety can harm your gut microbiome, from a therapist*. mindbodygreen. https://www.mindbodygreen.c om/articles/gut-health-mental-health-connection

15. Gis. (2021, June 1). *Your gut microbiota – balanced or not? - Gastrointestinal Society*. Gastrointestinal Society. https://badgut.org/information-centre/a-z-digestive-topics /gut-microbiota-balanced/#:~:text=Research%20shows%2 0that%20gut%20microorganisms,this%20state%20is%20cal led%20normobiosis

16. *Go with your gut: Gut health quiz*. Benenden Health. (2023, May 5). https://www.benenden.co.uk/be-healthy/body/g o-with-your-gut-quiz/

17. Goodreads. (n.d.). *The mind-gut connection quotes by Emeran   Mayer*.   Goodreads. https://www.goodreads.com/work/quotes/44319543-the

-mind-gut-connection-how-the-astonishing-dialogue-takin
g-place-in-ou

18. *Gut Health and nutrient absorption*. Ixcela. (n.d.)
. https://ixcela.com/resources/gut-health-and-nutrient-ab
sorption.html

19. *Gut health quiz*. The Gut Health Doctor. (2023, August 25).
https://www.theguthealthdoctor.com/gut-health-quiz

20. *Gut Stats & Gut Facts: All about gut health*. Pendulum. (n
.d.). https://pendulumlife.com/blogs/news/gut-stats-gut-f
acts-all-about-gut-health

21. Harvard Health. (2021, March 6). *Foods linked to better
brainpower*. https://www.health.harvard.edu/healthbeat/f
oods-linked-to-better-brainpower

22. *Inflammatory bowel disease clinic*. Support-
ed by the University of Alberta. (n.d.)
. http://www.ibdclinic.ca/what-is-ibd/digestive-system-an
d-its-function/why-is-digestion-important/

23. Jennings, K.-A. (2023, January 23). *11 best foods to boost your
brain and memory*. Healthline. https://www.healthline.co
m/nutrition/11-brain-foods

24. JHoldsworth. (2020, August 24). *The Gut Quiz*. Guts UK.
https://gutscharity.org.uk/2020/02/the-gut-quiz/

25. Kubala, J. (2023, June 16). *The 8 most common food intolerances*. Healthline. https://www.healthline.com/nutrition/
common-food-intolerances

26. *Lactose intolerance*. Lactose Intolerance | Boston Children's Hospital. (n.d.). https://www.childrenshospital.org/conditions/lactose-intolerance

27. Lauren Armstrong, R. (2020, July 14). *From food to poo: How long does digestion take?*. Greatist. https://greatist.com/health/how-long-does-it-take-to-digest-food

28. Makinde, S. (2023, April 17). *What are the signs of a healthy digestive system?*. Perfect Balance Clinic. https://www.perfectbalanceclinic.com/what-are-the-signs-of-a-healthy-digestive-system/

29. Mayo Foundation for Medical Education and Research. (2021, February 23). *Hiatal hernia*. Mayo Clinic. https://www.mayoclinic.org/diseases-conditions/hiatal-hernia/symptoms-causes/syc-20373379

30. Mayo Foundation for Medical Education and Research. (2022, April 28). *Relaxation techniques: Try these steps to reduce stress*. Mayo Clinic. https://www.mayoclinic.org/healthy-lifestyle/stress-management/in-depth/relaxation-technique/art-20045368

31. Mayo Foundation for Medical Education and Research. (2023, August 22). *Diarrhea*. Mayo Clinic. https://www.mayoclinic.org/diseases-conditions/diarrhea/symptoms-causes/syc-20352241

32. Mayo Foundation for Medical Education and Research. (2023a, January 4). *Gastroesophageal reflux disease (GERD)*. Mayo Clinic. https://www.mayoclinic.org/diseases-condit

ions/gerd/symptoms-causes/syc-20361940

33. Mayo Foundation for Medical Education and Research. (2023a, March 2). *Colon polyps.* Mayo Clinic. https://www.mayoclinic.org/diseases-conditions/colon
-polyps/symptoms-causes/syc-20352875

34. Mayo Foundation for Medical Education and Research.
(2023c, May 12). *Irritable bowel syndrome.* Mayo Clinic. https://www.mayoclinic.org/diseases-conditions/irrita
ble-bowel-syndrome/symptoms-causes/syc-20360016

35. Mayo Foundation for Medical Education and Research. (n.d.). *Lactose intolerance.* Mayo Clinic. https://www.mayoclinic.org/diseases-conditions/lactos
e-intolerance/symptoms-causes/syc-20374232

36. Mayo Foundation for Medical Education and
Research. (n.d.-a). *Gallstones.* Mayo Clin-
ic. https://www.mayoclinic.org/diseases-conditions/gallst
ones/symptoms-causes/syc-20354214

37. MediLexicon International. (n.d.). *Food intolerance: Causes,
types, symptoms, and diagnosis.* Medical News Today. http
s://www.medicalnewstoday.com/articles/263965#

38. MediLexicon International. (n.d.-a). *Common digestive disorders: Symptoms and treatments.* Medical News Today. https://www.medicalnewstoday.com/articles/list-of-d
igestive-disorders

39. Millar, A. (2021, November 1). *What's the link
between anxiety and Gut Health?* Patient.info

. https://patient.info/news-and-features/whats-the-link-be
tween-anxiety-and-gut-health

40. Northwestern Medicine. (n.d.). *Celiac disease vs. gluten intolerance (infographic).* https://www.nm.org/healthbeat/healthy-tips/celiac-disease-vs-gluten-intolerance-infographic

41. Novak, S. (2023, July 21). *Revealed: The five foods that are key to maintaining good gut health.* New Scientist. https://www.newscientist.com/article/2383723-revealed-the-five-foods-that-are-key-to-maintaining-good-gut-health/

42. Orenstein, B. W., Iliades, C., Fritz, A. L., Rapaport, L., Welch, A., Scott, J. A., Marks, J. L., Patino, E., & Rauf, D. (n.d.). *9 common digestive conditions from top to bottom.* EverydayHealth.com . https://www.everydayhealth.com/digestive-health/common-digestive-conditions-from-top-bottom/

43. Plevin, D., Galletly, C. The neuropsychiatric effects of vitamin C deficiency: a systematic review. *BMC Psychiatry* **20**, 315 (2020). https://doi.org/10.1186/s12888-020-02730-w

44. Polak K, Bergler-Czop B, Szczepanek M, Wojciechowska K, Frątczak A, Kiss N. Psoriasis and Gut Microbiome-Current State of Art. Int J Mol Sci. 2021 Apr 26;22(9):4529. doi: 10.3390/ijms22094529. PMID: 33926088; PMCID: PMC8123672.

45. professional, C. C. medical. (n.d.). *Digestive system: Function, Organs & Anatomy.* Cleveland Clinic. https://my.cle

velandclinic.org/health/body/7041-digestive-system

46. professional, C. C. medical. (n.d.-b). *Diverticulitis*. Cleveland Clinic. https://my.clevelandclinic.org/health/diseases/10352-diverticulitis

47. professional, C. C. medical. (n.d.-b). *Gastrointestinal diseases: Symptoms, treatment & causes*. Cleveland Clinic. https://my.clevelandclinic.org/health/articles/7040-gastrointestinal-diseases

48. professional, C. C. medical. (n.d.-b). *Gluten intolerance: Symptoms, test, non-celiac gluten sensitivity*. Cleveland Clinic. https://my.clevelandclinic.org/health/diseases/21622-gluten-intolerance

49. professional, C. C. medical. (n.d.-b). *Perianal abscess: Vs. hemorrhoid, causes & treatment, surgery*. Cleveland Clinic. https://my.clevelandclinic.org/health/diseases/23282-perianal-abscess

50. professional, C. C. medical. (n.d.-c). *Gastroparesis*. Cleveland Clinic. https://my.clevelandclinic.org/health/diseases/15522-gastroparesis

51. professional, C. C. medical. (n.d.-c). *Irritable bowel syndrome: IBS, symptoms, causes, treatment*. Cleveland Clinic. https://my.clevelandclinic.org/health/diseases/4342-irritable-bowel-syndrome-ibs

52. professional, C. C. medical. (n.d.-d). *Inflammatory bowel disease: Symptoms, treatment & diagnosis*. Cleveland Clinic. https://my.clevelandclinic.org/health/diseases/155

87-inflammatory-bowel-disease-overview

53. professional, C. C. medical. (n.d.-i). *Stomach cancer: Causes, symptoms, diagnosis & treatment.* Cleveland Clinic. https://my.clevelandclinic.org/health/diseases/15812-stomach-cancer

54. professional, C. C. medical. (n.d.-j). *What to know about the gut-brain connection.* Cleveland Clinic. https://my.clevelandclinic.org/health/body/the-gut-brain-connection

55. Rdn, C. C. (2024, February 26). *The secret of serotonin and gut health - My good gut. My Good Gut.* https://mygoodgut.com/serotonin-and-gut-health/

56. Robertson, R. (2023, April 3). *How does your gut microbiome impact your overall health?.* Healthline. https://www.healthline.com/nutrition/gut-microbiome-and-health

57. Rodrigues, F. G., Ormanji, M. S., Heilberg, I. P., Bakker, S. J. L., & de Borst, M. H. (2021). Interplay between gut microbiota, bone health and vascular calcification in chronic kidney disease. European journal of clinical investigation, 51(9), e13588. https://doi.org/10.1111/eci.13588

58. Sanchez, M. (2023, October 5). *What your poop says about your health.* HealthPartners Blog. https://www.healthpartners.com/blog/healthy-poop-chart/

59. Sarah. (2021, October 11). *8 lifestyle habits destroying your gut health.* Gut Performance. https://gutperformance.com.au/8-lifestyle-habits-destroying-your-gut-health/

60. Segula, D., Mwandiambira, V., Howson, W., & Allain, T. J. (2011). Case report--the 46 year old man with a 5 month history of vomiting. Malawi medical journal : the journal of Medical Association of Malawi, 23(2), 55–57. https://doi. org/10.4314/mmj.v23i2.70752

61. Sikora M, Stec A, Chrabaszcz M, Knot A, Waskiel-Burnat A, Rakowska A, Olszewska M, Rudnicka L. Gut Micro-biome in Psoriasis: An Updated Review. Pathogens. 2020 Jun 12;9(6):463. doi: 10.3390/pathogens9060463. PMID: 32545459; PMCID: PMC7350295.

62. Spend, E. (2022, June 28). Why you need prebiotics, probi-otics and postbiotics: The trifecta of good gut health. Body-Bio. https://bodybio.com/blogs/blog/prebiotics-vs-probi otics-vs-postbiotics

63. *Success stories*. Be Gut Happy. (n.d.). https://www.begutha ppy.co.uk/success-stories

64. *Success stories*. Heal Well Nutrition. (2021, June 13). https: //www.healwellnutrition.com/success-stories/

65. *Success story leaky gut health check– verisana labs*. Verisana. (2019, November 23). https://www.verisana.com/about-v erisana/success-story-leaky-gut/

66. Sussex Publishers. (n.d.). *The three channels of gut-brain communication*. Psychology Today. https://www.psychologytoday.com/us/blog/mood-by-micr obe/202307/the-three-channels-of-gut-brain-communicati on

67. Sydney Sprouse. (2022, July 20). *Your guide to how nutrients are absorbed by the body.* Ask The Scientists. https://askthe scientists.com/nutrient-absorption/

68. *Taking good care of yourself.* Mental Health America. (n.d.). https://mhanational.org/taking-good-care-yourself

69. *The brain-gut connection.* Johns Hopkins Medicine. (2021, November 1). https://www.hopkinsmedicine.org/health/ wellness-and-prevention/the-brain-gut-connection

70. *The Gut Brain Connection: How Gut Health Affects Mental Health - PsyCom.* The Gut Brain Connection: How Gut Health Affects Mental Health. (n.d.). https://www.psyco m.net/the-gut-brain-connection

71. *The gut-brain axis: How your gut affects your mental health.* CNET. (n.d.). https://www.cnet.com/health/nutrition/th e-gut-brain-axis-how-your-gut-affects-your-mental-health/

72. *The relationship between Gut Health and Anxiety.* KnowYourDNA. (2023, January 13). https://knowyourd na.com/gut-health-and-anxiety/

73. U.S. Department of Health and Human Services. (2018, October 16). *Gut communicates directly with brain.* National Institutes of Health. https://www.nih.gov/news-events/ni h-research-matters/gut-communicates-directly-brain

74. U.S. Department of Health and Human Services. (2022, July 15). *Gut troubles.* National Institutes of Health. http s://newsinhealth.nih.gov/2020/02/gut-troubles

75. U.S. Department of Health and Human Services. (2022b, August 8). *Emotional wellness toolkit*. National Institutes of Health. https://www.nih.gov/health-information/emotional-wellness-toolkit

76. U.S. Department of Health and Human Services. (n.d.) . *Your digestive system & how it works - niddk*. National Institute of Diabetes and Digestive and Kidney Diseases. https://www.niddk.nih.gov/health-information/digestive-diseases/digestive-system-how-it-works

77. U.S. Department of Health and Human Services. (n.d. -a). *Acid reflux (ger & gerd) in adults - niddk*. National Institute of Diabetes and Digestive and Kidney Diseases. https://www.niddk.nih.gov/health-information/digestive-diseases/acid-reflux-ger-gerd-adults

78. U.S. Department of Health and Human Services. (n.d.-a). *Your digestive system & how it works - niddk*. National Institute of Diabetes and Digestive and Kidney Diseases. https://www.niddk.nih.gov/health-information/digestive-diseases/digestive-system-how-it-works

79. U.S. Department of Health and Human Services. (n.d.-b). *Diverticular disease - NIDDK*. National Institute of Diabetes and Digestive and Kidney Diseases. https://www.niddk.nih.gov/health-information/digestive-diseases/diverticulosis-diverticulitis#:~:text=Diverticulosis%20is%20a%20condition%20that,call%20this%20condition%20diverticular%20disease

80. U.S. Department of Health and Human Services. (n.d.-b).

Gastroparesis - niddk. National Institute of Diabetes and Digestive and Kidney Diseases. https://www.niddk.nih.go v/health-information/digestive-diseases/gastroparesis

81. U.S. Department of Health and Human Services. (n.d. -b). *Symptoms & causes of celiac disease - NIDDK.* National Institute of Diabetes and Digestive and Kidney Diseases. https://www.niddk.nih.gov/health-information/dig estive-diseases/celiac-disease/symptoms-causes

82. *Ulcerative colitis case study.* Immunopaedia. (2022, December 5). https://www.immunopaedia.org.za/clinical-cases/gastroint estinal-disorders/a-case-of-persistent-bloody-diarrhoea/

83. Wang, R., Li, Z., Liu, S., & Zhang, D. (2023). Global, regional, and national burden of 10 digestive diseases in 204 countries and territories from 1990 to 2019. *Frontiers in Public Health, 11.* https://doi.org/10.3389/fpubh.2023.1 061453

84. Watson, S. (2020, April 1). *How long does it take to digest food?.* Healthline. https://www.healthline.com/health/ho w-long-does-it-take-to-digest-food

85. WebMD. (n.d.). *Anal abscess: Symptoms, causes, and treatments.* WebMD. https://www.webmd.com/a-to-z-guides/a nal-abscess

86. Wojtowecz, A. (2021, October 6). *What is the gut-brain axis? how gut health affects mental health.* Well.Org. https://wel l.org/healthy-body/what-is-gut-brain-axis/

87. *Your serotonin gut health connection*. Dr. Will Cole. (2022, August 30). https://drwillcole.com/gut-health/your-serotonin-gut-health-connection

88. Zhang, Y. J., Li, S., Gan, R. Y., Zhou, T., Xu, D. P., & Li, H. B. (2015). Impacts of gut bacteria on human health and diseases. International journal of molecular sciences, 16(4), 7493–7519. https://doi.org/10.3390/ijms16047493